BEYOND WORDS

Also by Swami Satchidananda
INTEGRAL YOGA HATHA

BEYOND WORDS

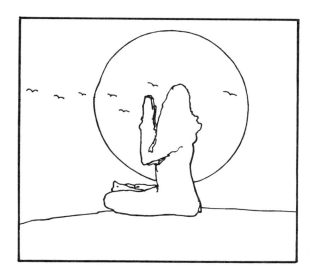

SWAMI SATCHIDANANDA

EDITED BY LESTER ALEXANDER
DESIGNED BY VICTOR ZURBEL
WITH THE DRAWINGS OF PETER MAX

Holt, Rinehart and Winston   New York

Published simultaneously in Canada by Holt, Rinehart
and Winston of Canada, Limited.

Satchidananda, Swami.
  Beyond words.

  1. Spiritual life (Hinduism)—Addresses,
essays, lectures. 2. Conduct of life—Addresses,
essays, lectures. I. Title.
BL1228.S27   294.5'44   76-29896
ISBN Hardbound: 0-03-020871-8
ISBN Paperback: 0-03-016911-9

First Edition

Printed in the United States of America
10 9 8 7 6 5 4 3 2 1

Preface

This book is assembled from the numerous transcribed lectures of Swami Satchidananda during the ten-year period 1966-1976. My goal was to present the essence of Swamiji's teachings in the clearest possible style without altering his meaning or editing out his personality. Where necessary, I have reconstructed and sometimes rewritten his words.

Swamiji gives so many public talks to so many different groups of people that he frequently repeats many of his favorite stories and thoughts. His basic point usually remains the same, but the flavor varies from telling to telling. I've selected many of these "favorites" and sometimes combined several different tellings into the one presented here.

This book by no means represents the totality of Swamiji's teaching. Those interested in going deeper into his work, may contact any of the Integral Yoga Institutes or the Satchidananda Ashram.

I would like to acknowledge Jennifer Josephy, my editor at Holt, Rinehart and Winston, for her tremendous support and weeks of concentrated time; Swami Hamsananda, for typing many of the original transcripts that I worked from; Swami Vidyananda, who lovingly reconstructed our first draft; Peter (Atman) Max, for the art that complements the words so perfectly; Victor (Arjuna) Zurbel, for the design that presents it so beautifully and the dedication that inspired me; and Patricia (Meera) Kerr along with my family and friends for their love and support.

Swamiji gave me the name Sukarta, meaning the one who does noble works and good deeds, and I offer this book to him as my thanks for bringing so much peace, love, happiness, and satisfaction into the lives of so many people.

Lester (Sukarta) Alexander
New York City
October 1976

Foreword

Absolute Truth is beyond the spoken or written word, beyond even the grasp of the finite mind. Still, we have to use words, even to say that the Truth is beyond them! So it is my sincere hope that these humble words will help the reader to go beyond the words to grasp the Spirit underlying them.

I sincerely wish to thank Lester (Sukarta) Alexander for the inspired and dedicated effort he has put into conceiving, editing, and bringing out this book, as well as Victor (Arjuna) Zurbel and Peter (Atman) Max for their beautiful design and artwork. I hope many readers will be benefited by the simple yet life-giving teachings of Yoga through this book.

Swami Satchidananda
Pomfret Center, Connecticut
August 1976

PEACE AND JOY
IS OUR GOAL

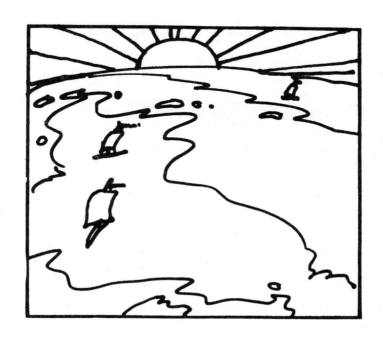

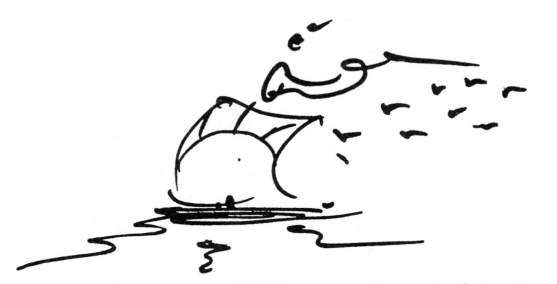

Peace and joy is our goal. Whatever we do, we are doing it for that. Not everyone believes in a God. But the real God, the absolute God, the cosmic God who is being searched for by one and all, is that peace and joy. Everyone wants that. Even the so-called nonbeliever or atheist, who would ignore the church or even burn down a temple, is after some peace and joy. He just feels that his actions will bring him that satisfaction.

If anybody asks me, "What is your philosophy or God?" I say, "Peace is my God." If they ask, "Where is He?" I reply, "He is in me and He is everywhere. He is all peaceful; He is all serenity. He is to be felt and experienced within oneself."

When you disturb your peace, you are denying the God within you. Money, drugs, position, whatever it be— anything that promises peace from outside will go one day. Nothing from outside can *give* you peace because peace is there in you, always.

There is a certain kind of deer from which we get musk fragrance. But that deer is always searching for the source of the fragrance. It doesn't realize that it comes from him; it is in him. Like that deer, we run here and there searching for that peace which is always within us.

We are peace personified, we are happiness personified, and when we miss that happiness, we want it again. In whatever we do, we are looking for that happiness. Can anybody ever say, "I'm doing all this because I want to be unhappy?" No. Even the man who wants to commit suicide wants to be happy by putting an end to his unhappiness. He is after that happiness even at the cost of his life.

Even if God Himself came and disturbed my peace, I would say, "Get away, I don't want You. I care more for my peace than for You." That is the way you must protect your goal. Don't allow anything to interfere with reaching that goal.

Once you reach it, all other things will come automatically, whether you want them or not. I never wanted ashrams and disciples; I never wanted publicity. I even ran away from all those things, but now they are running after me. Name and fame, praise and censure can come and go like passing clouds. But always remember the sun shining behind.

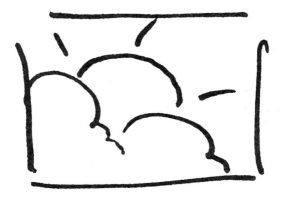

Don't be affected by circumstances. Just be simple and humble. If anything comes, scrutinize it; see whether it will help you move more quickly toward your goal. If so, take the help. Otherwise say, "No, I am not interested right now."

Once a King decided to test his ministers. He asked the ministers to bring many beautiful and valuable things to a park and arrange a big exhibition. They put a throne right in the middle and the King announced, "Before the sun sets, come and take whatever you want."

Everybody ran to the park and each one took something. But the condition was that they could not leave until the King gave the order to do so. Until then, they had to remain within the compound.

While everybody was picking and choosing, a peasant woman walked in. They all looked up to see what she would take. She walked over to the King and said, "Sir, I heard your offer. Are you sure you will give anything within the compound?"
"Yes, why do you question me?"
"I just wanted to make sure."
"Ask for anything you want."
"Well, Sir, I want you."

Everybody was shocked. "How dare she?"
The King said, "I, too, am inside the compound. All you people took my things but she took me. Yes, I'm yours, and so is everything that belongs to me."

That's what we should be doing with our inner peace. Seek that first. Don't run after tidbits, nibbling around here and there. If you really want something, want that and nothing less. Then you will get everything.

Beautiful parks, palaces, and music await you inside. Why go looking for these things outside? The entire Cosmos is within.

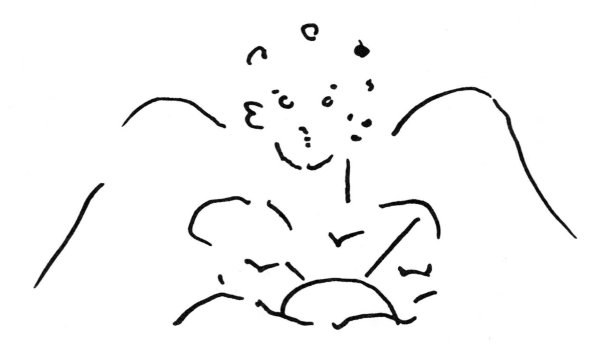

If you do not have peace within yourself you can never find peace outside. Once a businessman was talking seriously to a friend when his young son came and interrupted. To keep the boy occupied, the father found a world map, tore it into pieces, and gave it to the boy saying, "Son, will you please put them together again to form the world?"
The boy was really intelligent. He said, "Okay, I'll try."

He was a young boy who didn't know much about world geography, but he accidentally turned one piece over and saw a small bit of nose. Then he turned over other pieces and saw a hand, a leg, and a foot. He quickly turned all the pieces upside down and found different parts of the human body.

Very easily he arranged the body and then fastened it together and turned the whole thing over. Excited, he ran in to show his father. The father was surprised and asked how he did it.

"Oh, Father, it was very easy."
"The whole world was torn into pieces and you say it was very easy to put it together? How did you do it?"
"Daddy, I turned the pieces upside down and saw the parts of the human body, so I set right the human body and the world became all right."

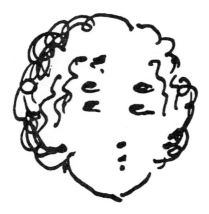

It is the same way in real life. To put the world together, you must first put the man together. If you want to see peace in the world outside, you must first see to it that your own mind is at peace. If you want to see a world free of greed, hatred, and jealousy, you must first see that your own mind is free of those qualities. As long as there are disturbances in your own mind, you will see disturbances in the world outside. So first put the man together and automatically you will be helping to put the world together.

Find the peace in yourself so that you can help others realize their own peace. That's not a selfish act. You are preparing yourself to serve. A razor must be sharpened before it is useful. Sharpening looks like a waste of time if you're in a hurry, but if you shave with a blunt razor, you will shave more skin than beard. Preparation is necessary for service.

For example, suppose a house is on fire and somebody is walking across the road with a bucket of gasoline. He sees the fire and says, "The house is on fire! I don't have time to go and exchange this bucket for one filled with water so let me throw the gasoline!"

I say it's better not to go near the fire. You aren't ready. If you don't have time to get a bucket of water, stay away. If you want to serve people, first become fit for such service by finding your own peace.

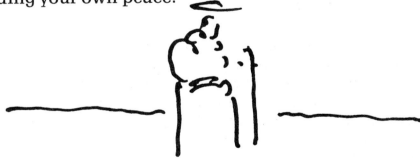

If you let an outside disturbance upset you, then you are the cause of your disturbance. If ten people are disturbed and you get upset too, you have not helped anyone and there is now one more disturbed person. Without getting disturbed, do something to make one person peaceful, then the ten will become nine. And the two of you can help two more and then there will be only seven.

I don't say you should sit quietly and do nothing. If so, I could easily have stayed in a cave somewhere in the Himalayas. Act, but retain your peace. The *Bhagavad Gita,* an ancient Yogic scripture, says to "see the inaction in action, and the action in inaction." When one part of you is well rooted in your peace, you can lend the other part to do some work for the benefit of humanity.

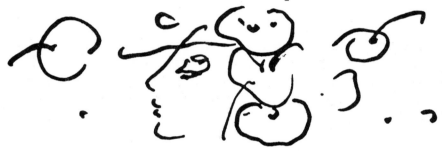

Your first duty is to find the peace in you. If you root yourself in your peace and then lend your hand, you will certainly bring peace. If not, you will only add more and more to the peaceless condition.

Violence cannot stop violence. A war can never really be won with violence alone. The mind must be changed. A violent victory only means that you have handicapped your enemy. He is still your enemy and the peace is only temporary. You have covered the fire so it doesn't show now, but it is still inside and one day it will flare up again.

When you win a war with your power, your enemy simply retreats and waits for an opportunity to strike back at you. You have won the war but not the heart. Real victory is to win the heart, not just the land or the political power.

Yoga tells you that your own peaceful thoughts will bring results. In the name of Yoga, we try to collect the mind and send out peaceful vibrations. A sincere thought will travel all over the world. It is more than an atomic bomb, it's more than a missile.

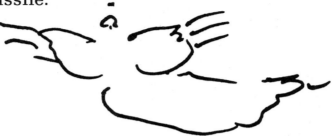

Even if you don't believe in God or prayer, sit and say, "Let there be peace. Let the minds of the people who want war be changed." We believe in thought force. Because it is the very same thought force that creates war. Remember that. It is the human mind that creates all these bombs, all these wars.

If you still want a war, fight it against undesirable thinking, not against a nation or people. And to fight such a war, you have to send out beautiful thoughts. Make every thought a powerful antimissile. Sit quietly and send out powerful, peaceful thoughts. I'm not joking—it is possible. Even one minute spent in peace is valuable. Don't think, "When our brothers are dying, how can we just sit quietly and think of peace?" This crazy world is, in a way, stabilized because of people sitting for a few minutes in meditation every day. Know that.

Don't ever think that by raising your hand or throwing a bomb or shouting something you can help the situation. Do it in a nonviolent way. Don't hurt anybody, don't hate anybody. As long as you have hatred in your mind, you are unfit to talk of peace.

How many great Emperors were there? Where are they now? Some are in history books. Some are not even there! But will the world ever forget the great spiritual Emperors, Jesus and Buddha? They achieved victory over the hearts of the people, not with ammunition but with the power of peaceful thoughts.

If we feel that the entire world belongs to us, how can there be a war? We are against evil, but not the evildoers. Let us produce beautiful vibrations so that all ugly thoughts will go away. This is the purpose of Yoga.

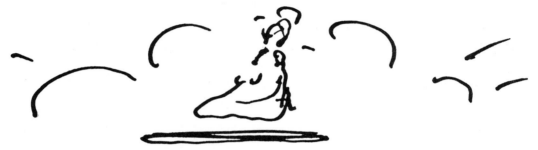

We work so hard for momentary pleasures. Imagine climbing Mount Everest. How much money and energy you must use! You climb and climb, so that when you reach the summit you can say, "I conquered." There's not even another person to hear you. You have only yourself to say it to. Why can't you just go and sit on the sofa in your own living room and say, "I conquered everything?" Nobody's going to question you.

Okay, you conquered Mount Everest. Can you build a home there? Can you even make yourself a cup of coffee? No. You just look around and then leave immediately. That is what I call momentary joy. I am not criticizing or condemning it. I'm just trying to show how much we pay for it, how much effort we put out, what elaborate preparations we make, how many years we work.

We are here to climb a peak, and what is its name? "Ever-rest!" Once you climb *that* peak, you don't need to come down. That is the difference between this Ever-rest and Mount Everest. Once you reach the abode of God, or peace, you remain there.

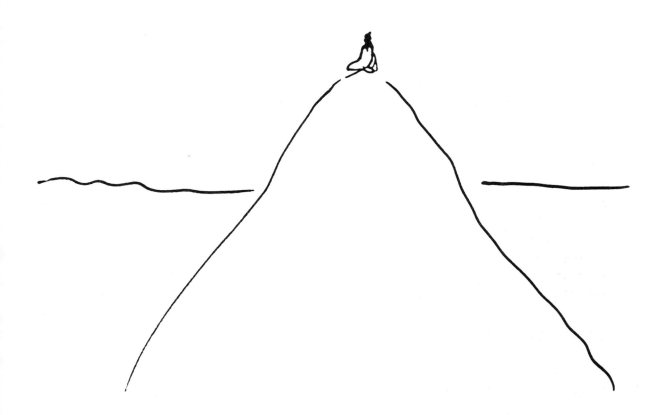

We all look for excitement, thinking that it is a plus. But what is a plus? A minus crossed.

A pendulum won't swing to the plus side and remain there. When it swings to one side, it automatically has to come back to the other. When you want excitement, and swing to that side, you naturally have to swing back to the other and you just keep on swinging. Then what do you call yourself? Swingers!

Nature's law is, the more you swing to one side, the more you swing back to the other.

The world has seen enough of that kind of excitement. Not that I say you should not swing. Go ahead, swing, but at least look up and see the other end of the pendulum. The upper end of the pendulum doesn't swing. It is fixed in one central place and remains there, well pivoted; that's why you are able to swing.

You can enjoy the swinging. We never say, "No, don't have any excitement; don't go to Miami or Las Vegas." Go ahead. Enjoy. But can you enjoy without disturbing your peace? If so, okay. It's a Yogic act because it is done without losing the center. If you don't lose the central point, you can swing along and really enjoy yourself.

Many of our lives are scattered instead of centered. We are on the circumference of a spinning wheel. The farther away from the center you are, the harder it is to balance. If you want to remain on the wheel and enjoy peace, where must you go? To the very center.

Real bliss is maintaining equanimity of mind at all times, at all places, under all circumstances, not only in church or synagogue, but in Times Square or on the battlefield. Closing your eyes and sitting in meditation isn't useful if you become useless as soon as you open your eyes. Real Yoga is applied equanimity, applied psychology, applied spirituality.

Don't get excited over profit or depressed over loss. In this life, we constantly face ups and downs, pleasure and pain, friendship and enmity. Some people praise you, some people curse you. We are constantly pulled and tossed between dualities.

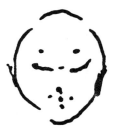

You see God in a baby's face because the baby's mind is calm, pure, and tranquil. A baby will as easily give a smile to a deadly enemy as to a close relative. It will play with a newspaper or a dollar bill, a piece of clay or a piece of gold. It looks at clay and gold, friend and enemy, rich and poor, profit and loss, as the same.

The world is a mixer. Wherever you see a right, there is a left. Wherever you see positive, there is negative. You can't just draw a line and say, "This is all good and that is all bad."

If you don't want a left wing, you should not have a right wing either. As long as you have a right wing, you are sure to have a left wing. So that is why we say neither go to the left nor to the right but come to the middle. It is on the middle path we find peace.

And yet, there's nothing wrong with the left or the right if we sit in the middle and use them properly. It's something like the two oars of a boat: both are necessary. If you always use one, you will just go round and round and round.

Every individual has a good and bad side. Even the so-called totally good man will have a little weakness somewhere. Otherwise he wouldn't be here in this world. It is that small percentage that is the anchor that hooks him here. He gets hung up. If he were one hundred percent good, there would be no hang-up and he would go up.

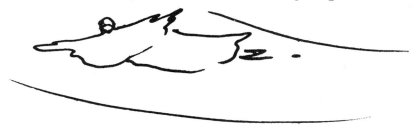

Forget about experiencing this and that and going here and there. Just be where you are. Enjoy the golden present. Do what is at hand. You are not going anywhere; you are not coming back from anywhere. We are where we are already, never going or coming.

Everything is an experience, so experience it. When you eat, experience what you are eating. When you work, experience what you are working at. And ultimately experience the experience itself. See the seer, hear the hearer, know the knower.

People with millions of thoughts in their minds sometimes can't even live happily for one minute on this earth. They want to go here, do this, do that, as if they have done everything that is to be done where they are. You are here now. Make this a heaven. You are in this town; make it heavenly.

Begin where you are. You don't need to look far away. Do that later, after you have improved your own place and surroundings.

You are all sparks of the divinity, images of God. You are nothing less than God Himself. You have that divinity, that goodness, that peace, and that perfect health. That is your true nature, so why should you run after anything?

Realize the God in you and make sure not to disturb it by wrong thinking or wrong actions. With this consciousness, you will spread peace and joy wherever you are.

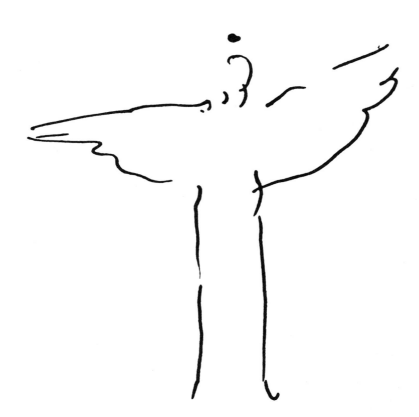

GOD

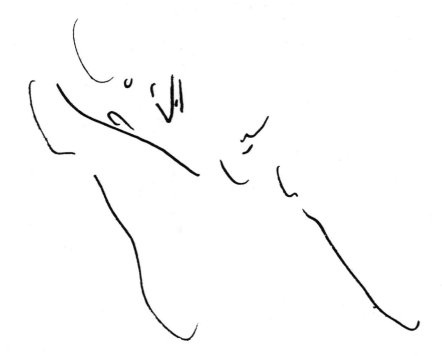

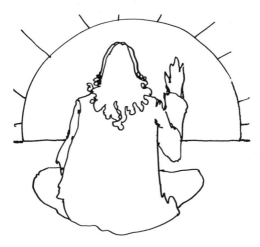

Ultimately, we are all seeking God, so we should know what God is. Suppose there is an apple sitting in front of you but you don't know what an apple is. You say, "I've never seen or tasted an apple. Perhaps there is no such thing!" If you don't know what an apple is, how can you know that you have one in front of you or enjoy its taste?

Suppose I give a talk for three hours about blueberry pie. Can you taste it? No. I will be wasting my time. Instead, I have to give you the recipe: one cup of this, a tablespoon of that; put this together, mix, and then put it all in the oven. But even that is not enough. You can't just take the recipe book, gold-gilt it, put it on an altar, wave incense, and say, "Blueberry pie, blueberry pie." You have to get the ingredients, cook them, and eat the pie.

You can get the recipe in five minutes. God gave a wonderful recipe in the form of the Ten Commandments. But many of us just put the Book on the altar or debate for hours on its meaning. How many have actually done the cooking and the eating?

God is not something that can be talked of. God must be experienced. The day man started talking about God, he created all kinds of religious fights and quarrels.

It is impossible for our limited minds to grasp the unlimited infinite One. So the finite mind takes a little part of the infinite that it can understand and says, "This is God for me." It's something like ten people going to the sea with ten different containers and taking some seawater.

If one goes with a bucket, he will get a bucketful of sea. If another takes a cup, he will get a cupful of sea. If your mind is bucket-sized, you have a bigger God. We limit the unlimited One to suit our limitations.

A limited, finite mind can't know the purpose of an infinite One. A small measuring instrument can't measure something immeasurable. Our understanding, our senses, and our mind are limited. The more you expand, the more you understand. But to understand the cosmic purpose fully, you must become a part of the Cosmic Consciousness. Once you become that, you understand it, but you won't come back to tell. It's something like a drop wanting to know how deep the sea is. It jumps in, but it can never come out to tell you because it becomes the sea.

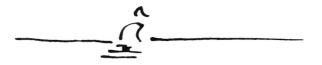

Before rain falls on the ground, it is tasteless, colorless, and odorless, but once it touches the ground, it assumes the color, odor, and taste of the earth. The same with our mind. When God is perceived through the mind, He takes the form of that mind. So each mind has its own conception of God. Everybody conceives of God according to his capacity, taste, and temperament.

The only thing we don't want is for people to fight about it. If there is a unity of understanding, there need not be a uniformity. There are as many religions as there are minds.

To understand God's way, we should become God. Real understanding is possible only when the person who says something and the person who listens come to the same level. God is pure and peaceful. When you become pure and peaceful, you will understand God by becoming Him. If you want your radio to receive a certain station, it should be tuned to the same wavelength as the transmitter. Then contact is made, the reception is perfect, and you hear music without any distortion.

If you want to understand God, tune yourself to God's wavelength. Until then, you cannot understand Him.

If a young girl, three or four years old, asks her mama, "Mama, how did you give birth to me?" the mama can answer with words, but she can never make the child understand how to give birth to a baby. For the time being, she says, "You jumped out of my stomach." When the child becomes a mother herself, then she really knows how her mama gave birth to her. It's a matter of experience. Until then, know that theoretical knowledge is just a limited understanding.

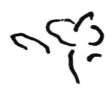

There was a man a long time ago who prayed every day, "God, I really want You to come in person, to have a nice sumptuous lunch with me."

Because he was constantly nagging, God appeared one day and said, "Okay, I'll come."
"God, I'm so happy. When can You come? You must give me some time to prepare everything."
"Okay, I'll come Friday."
Before He left, the man asked, "Can I invite my friends?"
"Sure," God said. And then He disappeared.

The man invited everybody and started preparing all kinds of delicious food. Friday at noon a huge dining table was set up. Everybody was there, with a big garland and water to wash God's feet. The man knew that God is punctual. When he heard the clock chiming twelve, he said, "What happened? God wouldn't disappoint me. He can't be late. Human beings can be late but not God."

He was a little puzzled but decided to wait another half-hour as a courtesy. Still no God. Then the guests began speaking, "You fool, you said God was coming. We had doubts. Why on earth would God come and eat with you? Come, let's go." The man said, "No, wait," and walked inside, to see what was happening.

To his great anxiety, he saw a big black dog on the dining table, eating everything there. "Oh, no! God sensed that the lunch was already eaten by a dog. That's why He didn't want to come." He took a big club and started beating the dog. The dog cried and ran away.

Then the man came out to his guests and said, "What can I do? Now, neither God nor you can eat because the food was polluted by a dog. I know that's why God didn't come." He felt so bad that he went back and started praying. Finally God appeared to him again, but there were wounds and bandages all over his body.

"What happened?" asked the man. "You must have gotten into a terrible accident."
"It was no accident," said God, "It was *you*!"
"Why do you blame me?"
"Because I came punctually at noon and started eating. Then you came and beat me. You clubbed me and broke my bones."
"But you didn't come!"
"Are you sure nobody was eating your food?"
"Well, yes, there was a black dog."
"Who is that, then, if not me? I really wanted to enjoy your food, so I came as a dog."

See? Everything is God. Don't look for God only in heaven or on the alter. Serve your dog. Serve your pigs. Serve the sick, serve the poor, serve the needy.

God made everything in His own image. God made the sky, the waters, the earth, everything. From what? If He made all these from a substance, from something, then my question is, "Who made that?" The only answer is God made everything out of Himself. Or, in other words, He Himself became the world. Know the world well and you will know God well.

If everything is God, then nothing is bad, nothing is good. It's all God. The very center of *God* is the letter *o*. It can mean nothing or everything.

But what is the use of an unmanifested God? He must manifest Himself in action. Current is everywhere, but what is the use? You have electricity wherever you have atoms, so why can't we just hold up a bulb and have it light up? Ramakrishna says, "Milk is everywhere in the body of the cow, but you can't pull at its ear and get milk, you have to pull at the udder."

It's the same with electricity; it is everywhere but you can't just get it anywhere you like. You have to get it through a generating station. When the dynamo moves, it gathers and collects the electricity and passes it to you through cables. If electricity doesn't express itself through a dynamo, it is of no use to us.

Mere existence is not enough. Express yourself. To use electricity, you need the right gadgets. If you want music, connect a radio. If you want light, connect a light bulb. If you want to cook food, connect an oven. If you want motion, connect a motor.

So what is the function of electricity then? What is its quality: hot, moving, vibrating, musical? By itself, it seems to be free from any quality. But it expresses various qualities according to the gadgets you connect.

If somebody says, "In our house the electricity always sings," another person will say, "No, no, in our home the electricity cooks." Electricity cannot do anything without gadgets. There is a difference in the gadgets but not in the spirit or the force behind them.

The current is the same everywhere. It is the cosmic current and there is only one generating station. It sends energy to us without wires. We are all the different gadgets. One sings, the other swings; one steals, the other catches him. The power that motivates the policeman and the robber is the same. The difference is in the gadgets. Don't think that all must become singers, or all must become any one thing. We need variety because each contributes to the other.

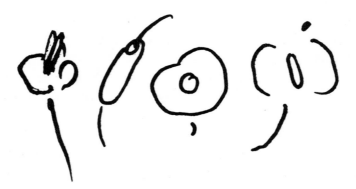

Some gadgets make better use of their power than others. Certain bulbs get the same voltage but give less light. What is the difference? In a 100-watt bulb, you have a longer filament than in a 60-watt bulb. The more you expand the filament, the more light you shed.

The heart is the filament here and the mind expands it. If you are a very narrow-minded person, you get only a little current. If you expand your mind more and more, you get more current and shed more light. That's why you should open up your heart. Don't be narrow. Then you get the current.

Once a man wanted to be away from the sun, so he said, "Go away, Sun, I don't want you." He closed all his doors and windows, sat in a dark room, and started cursing the sun. "I don't want to see you anymore. Don't come into my house."

He slowly opened the door and the sun started pushing in. He said, "No, no, get out," and slammed the door in his face. Then, after a while, he opened the door a little and again the sun came. He said, "What is this? Aren't you ashamed? Don't you have any pride? I am scolding you. Aren't you offended? Why don't you stay away? Why do you want to come into my house?"

The sun smiled and said, "That's my nature. If anybody opens the door, I just walk in. I don't need invitations. You can't push me out. You can't even invite me. All you have to do is open the door. I don't wait for your invitation and I am not offended by your scolding. All I need is an open door. You can't stop me."

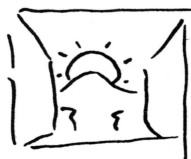

The sun shines on a holy church and on a lavatory. It shines on gutter water, it shines over pure water, it falls on everything. The sun knows no darkness. It is only we who know the darkness as well as the light. The light never knows darkness nor the darkness light. In the same way God never blesses anybody particularly. His nature is to bless everybody. You just open up and you see Him, that's all. All we need is an open heart.

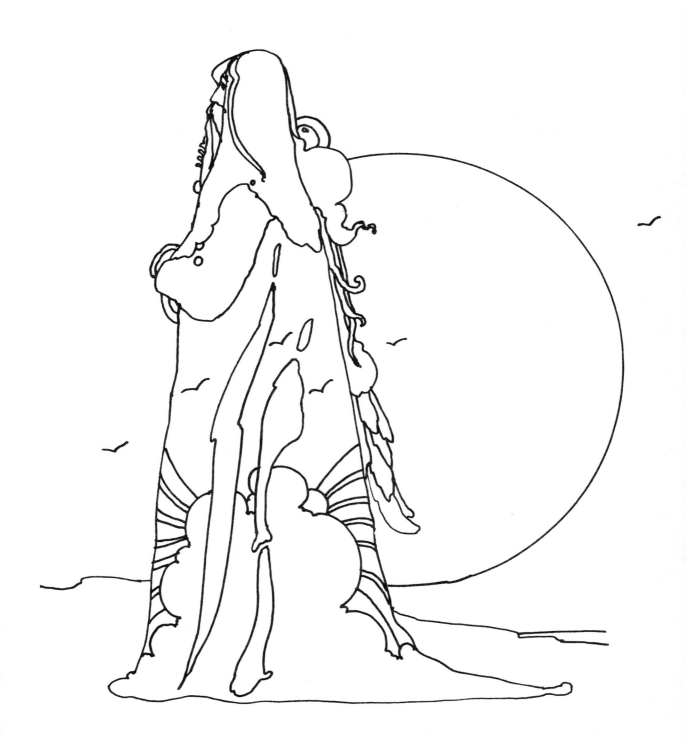

WE ARE ONE

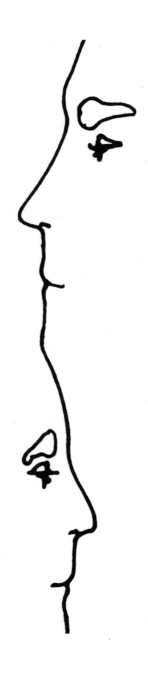

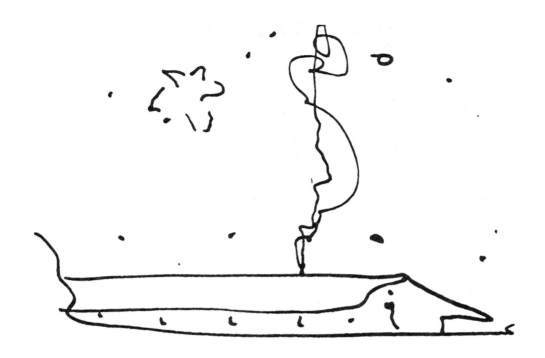

We don't eat the same food. We don't dress the same way or build our houses all the same. But we all eat, we are all dressed, and we are all sheltered. If I ask you why you eat, there is only one answer: to satisfy your hunger. But if I ask you *what* you eat, each one will probably give a different answer. Somebody will say, "I love Italian food." Another one will say, "I follow a macrobiotic diet." A third will say, "I like bread and butter."

Eat any food you want, call it by any name you want, shelter yourself anywhere you want, under the roof of a church, a synagogue, or the roof of the sky. It doesn't matter. Choose your own way, to suit your own taste, temperament, and capacity. There's no need to criticize or condemn those who follow a different path. Spiritual hunger is the same in all—the "food" to satisfy that hunger may vary.

If you are really hungry, do you bother to go and find a nice table with beautiful dishes to eat your food on? No. The moment you see a banana, you will peel and eat it even while you walk. You may not even wait to peel it! But if you take the banana and ask who produced it, who planted it, where it came from, and whether it was properly certified, you are not really hungry.

Divisions, differences, and varieties are necessary for enjoyment. If life is the same everywhere, it becomes monotonous. You get bored with the same food, the same people to see, and the same place to live. We get tired of it so we make things interesting. Sunday we eat Chinese food, Monday, Italian spaghetti, and Tuesday, macrobiotic. Variety is the spice of life.

But the real coming together can happen only when we rise above divisions and differences, when we see the variety but at the same time have that unifying vision. We create trouble when we leave out the unifying vision and see only the varieties.

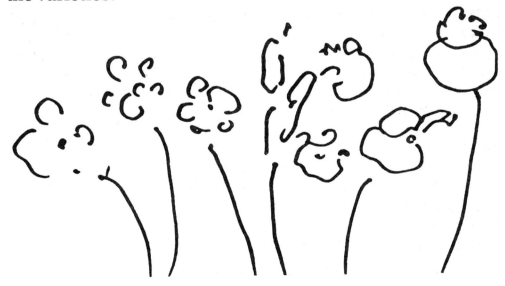

Imagine that the main wheel in a timepiece criticizes a small wheel saying, "You silly fellow, running so fast. Look how majestically I move."
Then the little fellow points to the balance wheel and says, "Well, look at *that* little fellow over there. At least I am better than he. He just goes one way, changes his mind, goes the other way, changes his mind, and goes back again."
"Yes, I see, you seem to be better than he!" And they both laugh at the balance wheel.

The little balance wheel listens carefully and then says, "Well, if you really make my work seem so little, so unreasonable, why should I do it? I'll strike." He stops and suddenly the movements of both the little and the big wheel stop with him.
The little one asks the big one, "Are you moving?"
"No. How about you?"
"No. How about the others?"
"We are all still."
"This calls for an urgent meeting."

Then the little fellow who had been moving this way and that laughs and says, "Now you know that we are all interconnected. We all do our own job. We have no individual purpose here. There is one common purpose for us all, to show the time. We are all equally important in our places. Who is great and who is small?"

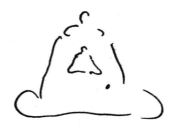

Nobody is inferior, nobody is superior. In the common plan, we are all just doing our part. We're all like pawns on a chessboard. Both the pawns and the queen are chipped from the same block of wood. Different pieces get different names. The minute they come onto the board, they get different movements. The queen says, "I can go anywhere I want!" What liberation she seems to have!

But all pieces are moved by the same hand. And they can only move while the play continues. Once the game is over, all return to the same box. And inside the box there's no king, no pawn, no bishop. There's no difference—just pieces of wood. If we keep this truth in mind and then play our part, the game is beautiful and we have Yoga.

And we'll be playing the game with all its rules, because there's no game without rules. You can't say, "Oh, we can move anywhere we want. The queen moves that way, why can't I?" If the bishop and pawn also want to move around like that, it's not a chessboard, it's a mess-board.

But that doesn't mean that we should lose our individuality. We still live as individuals but with the knowledge of our oneness. With this knowledge, we are one with the Cosmos, in Cosmic Consciousness, or whatever you want to call it, and that is what is meant by God.

In school, members of the same class will present a dramatic play at the end of the year. Each has a different costume. But behind all the different costumes they know that they belong to the same class. One person is made King and the other person is made the servant. After the curtain falls, if the King forgets the truth, that he and the servant are the same, and continues treating the other as a servant, there will be a fight.

In soccer, twenty-two people get together, then separate themselves into two teams, and even on each team every player has his own position. All have to stick to the rules of play, and if anybody fouls, he is penalized. He may say, "It's all in fun, what's the harm in fouling?" It's fun, no doubt, but it disrupts the game. It's not fun for the other players then.

To have a game, you have to play within the rules, and that is what we are doing in this life. We are all playing the game. Each one is supposed to play his part well. We all came here together and separated ourselves for the sake of play, like fullbacks, halfbacks, and goalkeepers.

The entire globe is our playground. We have a set of rules—the moral precepts—and our own roles to play. If a person remembers this, he will play his part beautifully without inconveniencing others. But if even one person in the game constantly makes fouls, the play gets interrupted.

Everyone has a responsibility. No one should think that he is insignificant and that without him the world can carry on. Nobody is unwanted or undesirable here. Know that positively. As in a machine, every screw, every nut, and every bolt is indispensable. If even one screw gets loose, will the machine run properly?

Don't think, "What on earth can I do? I'm not a prophet. I'm a puny little thing." If you were that puny and unwanted, God would not have created you and given you food and earth and air. You are the equal of anybody in this world.

The very fact that you are still living means that God has some work for you. You have a mission to fulfill, and you are doing it, whether knowingly or unknowingly.

You are not just an individual but a part of the whole. There is a cosmic plan; allow it to happen through you. There is one director; you are all the actors. You have been given a costume and are enacting your part. Until the curtain falls, you have no choice. You cannot change the story while you are on the stage. That is the ultimate understanding.

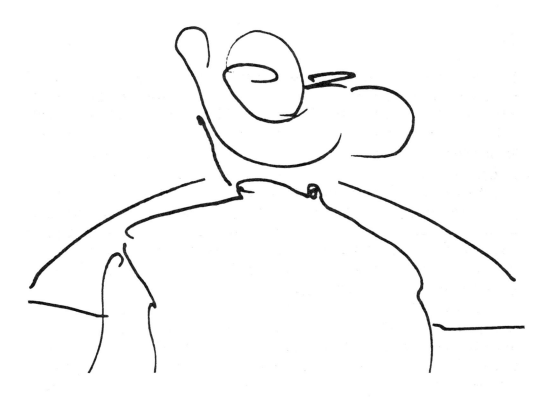

Every house has some essential parts, a foundation, floor, walls, and roof. Without them, there's no house. What is nonessential? The decorations, the gardens outside, the plants, light fixtures, and draperies. They vary because you decorate to suit your taste. If all houses were the same, it would be very boring. But you don't get bored if you see walls, a foundation, and a roof because you know they are necessary.

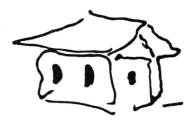

Religion also is like that. And the fundamental part is what we call Yoga. We don't worry about the superficial things. That we leave to you. We give you some examples, with different designs. Choose any design you want, or create your own.

"Hinduism," "Catholicism," and "Judaism," all the "isms" are different decorations. But they all have the same basic principle, that the individual must become fit to realize the Cosmic One, to know that he is not different from the Cosmic One. Let us accept all the different paths as different rivers running toward the same ocean.

Though we talk of the Cosmos and ourselves as being separate, we belong to it. We are within it. Without drops of water there is no ocean. An ocean is drops of water put together. So we are all drops, but we treat ourselves as individuals, as separate from other persons, losing sight of the Cosmic Truth and fundamental oneness.

The purpose of religion, or Yoga, is to realize that oneness. How? By refining the individual. The ignorance that makes us feel separate from others is to be removed. Fill up a balloon with air until it bursts. The balloon is only a temporary partition that divides the inner air from the outer air. Once the feeling of individuality or ego is broken, you are there as a whole, as a universal being.

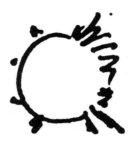

One day, I was working in the field and I hurt my finger. I could have ignored it, but I cleaned and bandaged it. If I had ignored it and the finger got infected, my entire body would have suffered. The same way, if we feel we are parts of the cosmic body—the entire universe—how can we stop from loving the other parts? We're not separate from anyone. It is our duty to love and take care of our world.

The head that thinks it need not worry about an infection in the thumb because the thumb is different will get the infection itself very soon. Once you feel that you are a part of the whole, that you belong to the whole and the whole world belongs to you, that very feeling makes you love, and that very love brings forth healing vibrations from you. You need not even touch or see people, you just think of them. By your mere thinking, you send healing vibrations. No healer can heal without that universal love.

If you realize that you are not just an individual but a part of the whole universe, you will not be afraid of anyone. A fearless man lives always, a fearful man dies every day, every minute. And you will never feel loneliness. You are always with people, with your work, with your activities. And your own conscience, which is a part of God, is always with you.

People oftentimes feel loneliness when they miss some particular individual with whom they want to be close. They are attached to some thing or person. Sometimes they feel lonely even in the midst of a gathering of many people. You need not depend on one individual. Learn to appreciate the good company of your own feelings, of the God in you, and the joy of the service you are performing.

Loneliness should be properly understood. It is in the mind. It is a feeling of lacking something. Think of all that you have. Then you will feel, "I am surrounded by so many people, so many things, beautiful flowers, land, plants, everything." Communicate with a flower. It is already smiling at you. Real communion with God is communion with your fellow beings.

Let us feel that we are the children of that One Father or the One Creator. We're all interdependent, links in the same beginningless and endless chain, cells of a huge universal body. We are all One.

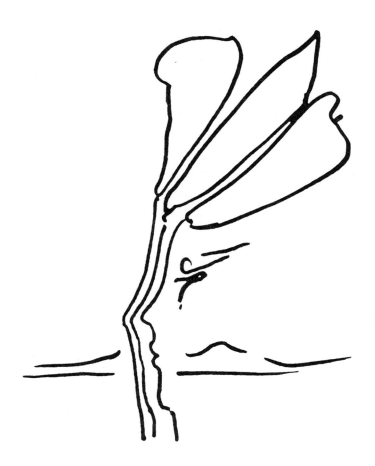

HE AND HIS ART
MAKE THE HEART

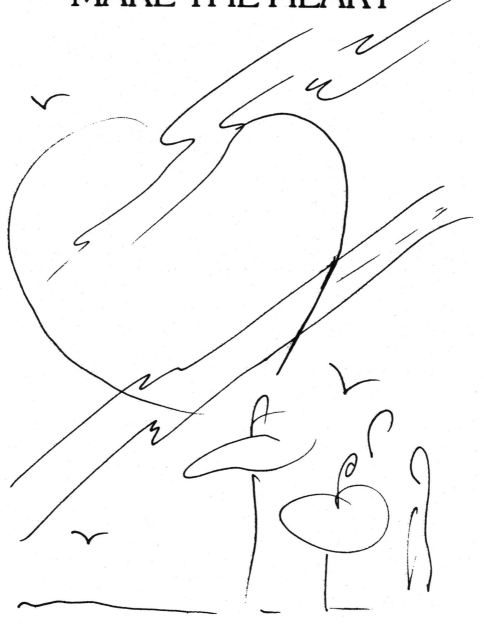

HE + ARY = HEARY

He and His *art* make the heart. *He* and His *ad* make the head. The head is only an advertisement. It is the ego looking for recognition.

We can never become one in the head, but we can come closer in the heart. Hearts are soft and tender and understanding. When two lovers come together, they address each other as "sweetheart," because the heart is sweet.

Have you ever heard anybody say "my sweethead"? Never. The head can never be sweet. That doesn't mean we should cut it off. It should be there, but let feelings take the lead, and the head will follow.

Yoga goes down to the heart to make everything a Yogic art. It tells us to go in a little to see the heart. Then, from that level, we can function through the head. Look within. The kingdom of God is within you. The name for God in Tamil, a South Indian language, is "go in."

Real marriage is when two people agree on one goal or purpose in life. God has given us two eyes to see as one. In the same way, as husband and wife you are two but you should see as one. The two minds are the two eyes. You should have one goal and toward that goal you should both go like the two wings of the same bird or two oars of the same boat.

If your minds do not agree on one goal, then there's no marriage at all. You're simply living together for your convenience. When that common goal ceases to exist, so does the marriage. Then, instead of living together, constantly fighting and going off in different directions, it's better to say, "You take your life and go your way, I will go mine." There's nothing wrong in doing that. It's much better than living in the same house and constantly disturbing each other. If you have different aims in life, each should have the freedom to choose what he or she wants.

But at the same time, if you have children, I suggest that you wait and adjust as much as possible, for the sake of the children. Even if you have different goals, you both have a certain duty toward the children.

Sometimes, when you are living together with the same goal and purpose, there still may be a little friction now and then. That kind of friction is good because life is dull when it is always smooth. A little pinching here and there is okay. I don't say that a marriage should always be like milk and honey. If there is no friction for a whole week, give a little pinch! But it should not continue for long.

If a quarrel begins in the morning, it should end with lunch. If it begins at noon, it should end in the evening. Food without salt is tasteless; food with excess salt is also no good. A little bit of friction, like salt, will enrich your togetherness. But forget not that you have one goal—to progress, to evolve more and more, and to express your divine identity.

Feel that you are divine beings within. Help each other to refine yourselves. Live like god and goddess. That is why you take a vow of living together in the presence of God.

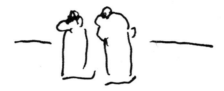

You don't need to live a celibate life if you don't want to. But set limits. Sexual energy, when stored, will build the brain and nerves. So, for the preservation of that vitality, you should limit your sexual life.

Yoga is only against overindulgence. Yoga is neither for the man who eats too much nor the one who fasts excessively, for the person who sleeps a lot nor the one who forgoes all sleep. That means finding a middle path. Neither suppress nor overindulge. Live with your partner, enjoy yourself, and if you wish, and can support them, have a few children.

From conception, the mother molds her child. Don't think that a child's education begins only after birth. The mother's very thinking is absorbed by the child within.

That's why a woman who is pregnant should read inspiring, holy books, no shocking novels or crime stories. If she wants the baby to be a great hero, she should read books about such people. If she wants a saintly person, she should read stories about the saints.

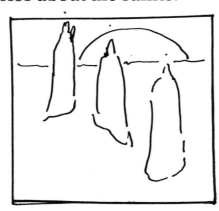

Today, I come across many girls who want to be mothers. Fine, but if you really want to be a mother, prepare yourself. Bringing forth a new life into the world is a great responsibility. If you are not fit, it's better not to have a child. A child is not a plaything. If you want a plaything, there are many beautiful plastic toys.

Bringing forth children and teaching them is a big task. Don't think that it's an easy thing. If you don't have the patience, if you can't give the time, if you are more interested in your own social life, then don't give birth to babies. They are not machines. You can't just bring them into the world and put them in a corner or employ somebody to take care of them while you go off with your tennis racket.

No. You have to sacrifice your time and energy for the sake of that soul. In the name of Western civilization you do many things that are totally unnatural. You don't even give your babies the food God prepared in your breasts. You want to go to a movie and pay a baby-sitter. If you are that interested in the cinema, you should not have brought forth a baby.

It gives me such pain to think about it. Many children are neurotic nowadays because of their parents' attitudes. Don't think money alone will bring peace and joy. The child doesn't want your material things. It wants your love and proper discipline.

How many of you were starved for love by your own parents? It is this that has created so many mental and social problems in this country—no love in the home, no love in the church, no love in the schools.

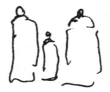

Express your love for your parents; don't be afraid of it, and listen to them. If there is some sense or proper guidance in what they say, accept it, because they are telling you for your own sake. Of course, sometimes parents don't want to understand what you are doing. Take, for example, spending your vacation in an ashram. Parents say, "A Yoga ashram? What is this Yoga? Don't even tell me. Come, let's go to Miami. You can sunbathe and there'll be lots of people to have fun with."

If what they're saying comes from their attachment to you, and what you are going to do is really beneficial to you or has benefited many other people, just tell them, "I'm going. Wait and give me some time. See if I'm wrong or if something terrible happens. If so, I'll come back."

But if they scold and abuse you and it is really too much for you to bear, know that the whole world is your father and mother. You don't need to hate your parents, just leave and go wherever you can find peace.

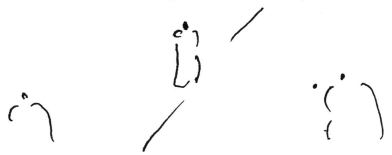

I am the last person to tell a child to leave his parents. But if parents can't understand their child, they are no longer parents. They are not interested in their child's welfare. By living with them, you are not growing and they are not being helped by you. So it's better to stay away, and perhaps one day, when they see you are growing well and are happy, they may come to you. Many a parent has told me, "I totally disapproved of my child, but now I see that what he is doing is good. I made a mistake."

In any case, if you are interested in Yoga, you should remove hatred from your heart. You cannot grow with poison in your mind, even if you think your parents are the cause of it. In a way, you are also the cause, because you haven't properly understood them. They may be doing something wrong, but if they knew it was wrong, they wouldn't do it.

Sympathize with them. Sincerely pray for understanding to grow between you. Love them more and never hate them. That's Yoga. Yoga never wants to separate anybody. Its interest is in bringing the whole world together. And sometimes the parents become better Yogis than the children!

A father should always forgive his son. A friend should forgive another friend, and a lover should always forgive his beloved. It is in forgiveness that you show your true affection. Any man can seek revenge but it takes a King or a Prince to grant a pardon.

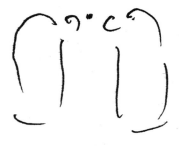

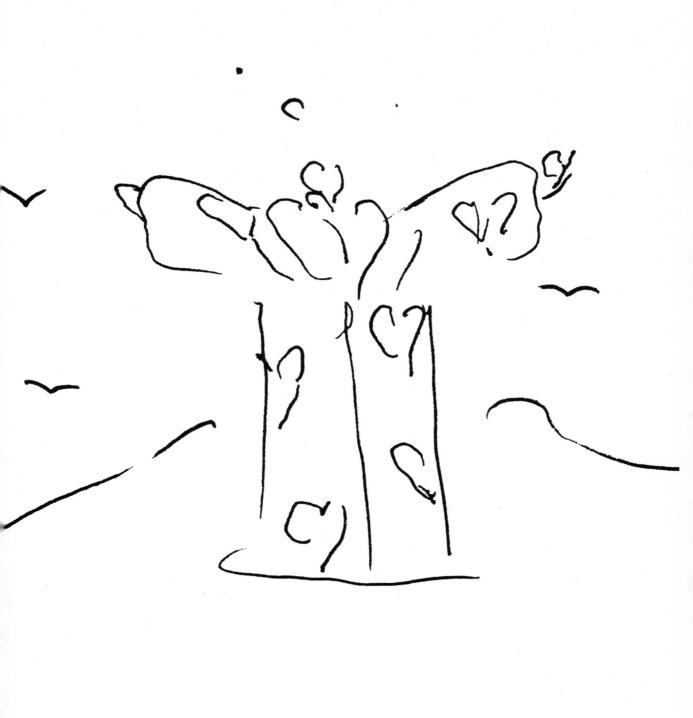

BODY AND BREATH

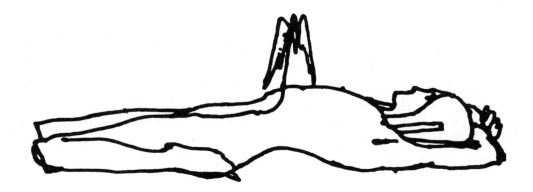

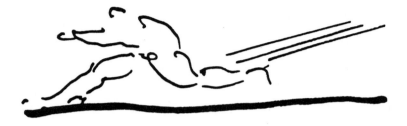

While we are here in these bodies we should know that they are vehicles of divine expression, as are all forms of Creation. We have to take care of the body because without a healthy one, nothing is possible in this world, either spiritual or material. To become a good instrument of the Divine, maintain your health, have an easeful body, a peaceful mind, and a useful life.

We can live without food for some time. We can live without water for some time, but we cannot live without breath. We breathe about fifteen times a minute. If the air leaves without returning, we die. Every time it leaves, we are about to die.

Do we consciously draw it back when it leaves? No. We are not even conscious of breathing. There is an unseen force that takes care of us and causes the air to return. You may say, "Swami doesn't seem to know much about anatomy. There are sets of muscles, voluntary and involuntary, and when the chest cavity expands, a vacuum is created. The breath returns to fill up that vacuum."

To such people I say, "Who makes the chest cavity expand? Do you? Can you keep it from expanding, or can you keep it from contracting after expansion?" No. You have a say over it for a maximum of a few minutes, and afterward, the involuntary muscles take over. That's why you call them "involuntary." The moment you use the word *involuntary*, you accept that it is not in your hands. Something or somebody is doing it.

Who is that somebody? I say it is the One who sent you here, the One who extracts some work from you, the One who takes care of His plans through us all.

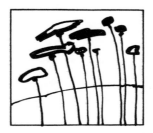

Somehow, a baby knows it is coming into this crazy world and that's why it arrives crying, "God, why are You sending me into this asylum? What have I done to You?" As he comes out crying, we laugh and celebrate.

And toward the end, it's the other way around. When he gets liberated and walks out happily, we cry.

What is it that is young or old? It is the body. You were never born and you are never going to die. You are ageless; only the body has ages. The soul knows itself to be unlimited and immortal. It is that immortality which we should realize.

The worst fear is the fear of death of the body. When your old clothes wear out, you throw them away and put on new ones. We all have old-model bodies. We will get new ones, don't worry. After all, how long are you going to live in this body? Maybe another fifty or sixty years.

All our burial grounds are nothing but junkyards. There's no need to be afraid of death. Laugh at it. The man who is afraid of death dies every day but a hero dies only once. Let death come once to us. Be bold and proud.

Death means change of form, that's all. It is inevitable and it is happening every minute. You are not the same person you were a minute ago. A part of you is already dead and a part is being born.

The soul simply changes vehicles. When the tree dies, you get planks. When the planks die, you get a chair. When the chair dies, you get firewood. When the firewood dies, you get ash.

Nothing can really be destroyed; we just change names and forms. There is no death at all. What is, is always. What is not, is not, and will never be. What you call the world is nothing but ever-changing names and forms.

We say this is cloth, but is it really cloth? What you see is cotton twisted into threads and woven and arranged in the particular way you call cloth. If I disperse the arrangement and heap the threads into one pile, the cloth vanishes.

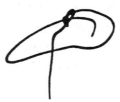

I didn't destroy anything. I disturbed the arrangement of the threads, that's all. So if you say you see cloth, it is a falsehood. That is how we live a false life in this world. We never speak truth in its real sense. Everybody is a liar here, including me. And even when I say everybody is a liar, that itself is a lie!

Nothing is ugly in its natural state. A rose is beautiful, a dog is beautiful, a pig is beautiful, everything is beautiful in its own way. In trying to *make* things beautiful, we cover their own natural beauty. Babies' faces have cosmic beauty which slowly becomes hidden by ugly thoughts and habits. Then we try to make the face beautiful again artificially and call that cosmetic beauty.

To beautify themselves, some women do all kinds of unnatural, artificial things which can make them sick. In the name of beauty, they apply all kinds of powders and creams. Their pores are totally blocked. There's no perspiration and all the secretions that should come out go back into the bloodstream. A cotton dress will absorb perspiration but nylon and synthetic materials can't. There is no ventilation so when you perspire it doesn't get absorbed by the air outside and it goes back into the system.

Many people don't think it's fashionable to sneeze or cough. Don't let "civilized" habits stop the body's natural elimination. You cause great damage to the body and affect hundreds of nerves by controlling your sneezing and coughing. When you sneeze, God will bless you.

Take care of your intake, physical and mental. Be careful what goes in. Every country has its immigration office. Before somebody walks in, they ask, "Who are you? Friend or foe? What are your credentials? Show us your passport. If you are a good person, be our guest. If not, get out."

Your body is your country and there are many ports of entry. You should put immigration officers everywhere.

Much of what we call civilization is artificial and unhealthy. We must return to natural living. That is Yoga.

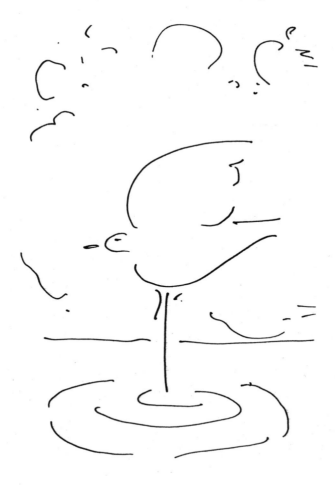

Go to the zoo and watch the animals. All the carnivores seem to be restless, prowling around even within their cages. Then watch the vegetarian animals. They are so soft and gentle. They look at you and smile.

Animal fat leaves more toxins in the system than vegetables and is not conducive to a peaceful mind. Animal food is dead matter. Anything that is dead will immediately start decomposing and be unfit for eating. When you cut a piece of flesh from a body, it decays, whereas a vegetable is still a living organism. Take a potato, eat half of it, cut the other half into ten pieces, plant them, and you will get ten potato plants. Take a goat, eat one half, make ten pieces of the other half, plant them, and tell me what you get. A bean has life in it after several months. Some seeds have life in them even after hundreds and thousands of years.

You get enough protein in an easily assimilable form from seeds, beans, grains, milk products, and vegetables. The energy that you waste in digesting meat is more than you gain from it and it takes a long time to digest. That's why you have to cook meat so long. If it is left undigested, it starts decomposing and fermenting in the system.

Eat foods that are fresh, alive, and not overly cooked. Try to avoid eating stale leftovers. Prepare enough for one meal and finish it.

Another reason we follow a vegetarian diet in Yoga is because we do not wish to kill any developed conscious life for our sake. Every time you eat something, you kill something, no doubt. But it is the violence, the pain that you cause to animals that we wish to avoid. If you never eat meat or kill any animals, the animal kingdom all over the globe will worship you. Wherever you are, they will sense that you are a person of nonviolence and a good friend.

Food is from Nature, air is from Nature, and water is from Nature. We take things from Nature, so we have to return things to Her. We cannot return exactly what we take, but we can convert the food, the air, and the water into energy and utilize that energy for the benefit of the world. Then we are not debtors.

Whatever you eat is Mother Nature in the form of food. The fruits are your mother, the grains are your mother, the whole earth is your mother. So we say, "Mother Nature, in the form of food, let me have you. And by this, let me have wisdom, dispassion, and health. And when I have strength, and health, and dispassion, let me be a better person, a useful person." This should be our purpose in eating.

Many people, when they get worried, pour a drink, take something to get high, or go to the refrigerator. What are they actually doing? They don't remove the cause of the worry or the problem, they only push it under the rug. Have you ever seen an animal smoking or drinking? No. We become worse than the animals when we do these things.

A shot of whiskey or a joint won't help you find the cause of your disturbance and eliminate it. You were not born restless. You were born with peace and, by your own wrong actions, have disturbed it. When you say somebody is diseased, you mean that he has lost his natural ease. He had ease, he "dis-turbed" it, so now he has "dis-ease."

If a frightening thing is coming toward you and you don't know how to avoid it, you can simply close your eyes. The danger seems to go away but you have not really removed it. We do this in many, many ways. When there is a headache or stomachache, we don't try to find the cause. Why should the head ache all of a sudden? What went wrong? We never think of that but immediately take an aspirin.

We do this much too often in our daily life; we swallow something to temporarily forget the worry. But once the intoxication is over, we wake up with the same problem, only worse, because the force that we applied to cover it up has weakened our system.

How can a drug keep the mind clean and calm when it only adds more dirt? Temporarily, it makes you forget the disturbed feeling. It's something like an induced sleep. A sleeping pill will make you feel that you are sleeping but it's not real sleep. A tranquilizer will make you feel that you are tranquilized but it's not true tranquility. It's only a temporary feeling.

Pain is caused by some trouble. When you take a painkiller, an injection, or a pill, you don't feel the trouble. Does it mean that you have cured the trouble? Not at all. It's something like cutting the wires of a fire alarm. It will stop the alarm immediately, but it won't put out the fire. Pain is your fire alarm. When the body is on fire somewhere, the pain says, "There's trouble." Find the cause of the trouble instead of finding ways to cover it up.

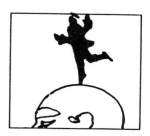

The body and the mind are interconnected and interdependent. The body expresses the thoughts of the mind. Constantly thinking crooked thoughts will create a crooked body. If you have a happy mind, your face and body will reflect that happiness. Everybody will know something beautiful is happening within you.

Suppose I take a small packet, open it, and say, "It's some very delicious candy." Without my even showing you the candy, you may salivate. The mind hears the sound "candy" and the body reacts. Suppose somebody shouts at you, "Hey, you stupid fool!" You will get angry. When you are angry, the blood boils and the face becomes red. You only hear a sound but your mind gets angry and makes your body react.

Here's a different example. You are a singer ready to give a performance and all of a sudden you feel a pain in your stomach. Can you sing with joy? No. Just as mental pain affects the body, bodily pain affects the mind.

Suppose a man who is always happy and joyful falls sick. He has a high fever and lies in bed. One day he feels very thirsty and asks his son to get him a drink of water. The child is delayed and returns half an hour later with the water.

Normally, he would smile at the child and forgive him. But because he is weak and ill, he gets irritated and starts shouting at him. A sick man gets irritated quickly because the body is weak.

When the mind and body are weak, you don't have the capacity to avoid bad habits. Cravings and desires will bother you. Never suppress any desire. Instead, develop a better desire. Then you won't have time to respond to the original one.

Don't force yourself to get rid of a bad habit. Forcing yourself is something like beating the darkness with sticks. You can walk into a totally dark room with some friends and begin beating the darkness with sticks shouting at it to leave. Hundreds of people can beat the darkness for hours and it will still remain.

The sensible man will just light a candle and bring it into the room. Yoga is that candle. Bring it into your life and all your unwanted habits will leave. You need not bother yourself about them. When the mind and body are strong, they will just drop away.

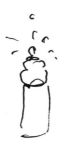

This is the reason for practicing the physical postures that we call the Yoga *asanas.* Putting your body in the different positions builds up strength within the system. You tone the muscles, organs, endocrine glands, spine, and all the nerve centers. The asanas do not cause strain like many other exercises. They are done very gently, with grace and ease.

Another important practice is breath control or *pranayama.* By proper breathing, you learn to use the entire capacity of the lungs and you charge the system with extra oxygen and vitality.

As you start doing these practices, you gradually strengthen the physical system. And because you do them in a gentle way, you help calm your agitated mind. Whenever you are tense, worried, or bothered, just take a few slow, deep breaths through the nose with full attention and you can easily calm the mind. If you regulate the breath, you have regulated the mind. In the same way, if you regulate the mind, you can regulate the breath.

Through Yoga, you are trying to control your inner nature, which is governed by your vital energy or *prana.* Prana is our very life, the absolute force which is present and functioning everywhere. We can live for many weeks without food, days without water, minutes without air, but not even for a fraction of a second without prana.

The best way to control the prana is to control the breath, and when you have mastery over the prana, you have gained mastery over your inner nature. Every act or thought is the expression of the subtle movement of the prana in the system. By controlling the prana, you control the thought, and vice versa.

There is a kind of lamp that has a plain light bulb inside with a multicolored cylinder around it. Around the colored cylinder is a plastic sphere with many diamond-shaped facets. The heat of the bulb makes the cylinder rotate around it, throwing light of many different colors onto the sphere, which then projects a moving pattern of colored light into the room.

The stationary bulb is like the True Self. Its light is constant and stationary. It shines and produces heat, which is like your dynamic energy or prana. The colored cylinder is made of plastic and is slightly twisted. Because of these twists, it absorbs the heat from the bulb unevenly and starts revolving. So, too, the mind and the ego have lots of twists and holes. The heat from the True Self makes them spin around and around, throwing out different colors.

The colors we see projected into the room do not belong to the bulb, they belong to the revolving cylinder. Suppose you remove all the facets from the sphere and make it smooth, then remove all the colors and twists from the revolving disk. Now, even though the bulb creates heat, the cylinder won't revolve; it will just throw pure light outside.

If the plastic cylinder is kept from revolving, it will get very hot and burn up. If you make the ego clear and pure and remove all the colors and twists, it too will slowly burn up. So, to allow your True Self to shine out, you should see that the revolving cylinder, which is your individual nature, is purified and made still. A person who has controlled his inner nature can allow his true light to shine outside. That is why you see something special in him and call him a holy man. It's not that he alone has holiness—everyone has—but when we do not have this kind of control, our light shines out in different, distorted ways.

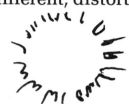

Purification and control of the prana can be attained in several ways. Whatever method we use, the ultimate goal is to control our inner nature, to make it clean and calm, so that the divine light within can be seen by everyone. That is why we need discipline. Without discipline, you can't calm anything. Discipline means you regulate things, you make them run in a harmonious, rhythmic way.

Imagine you are tied to the saddle of a galloping horse, clinging for your life, hoping that somehow the horse might feel sympathy and stop. Is that enjoyment? The man who really enjoys horseback riding is the one who controls the horse, who can stop whenever he wants.

In that sense, you can enjoy anything you want. Nothing is dangerous then. If you want to drink, drink. But can you stop whenever you want and stay away for months and months without even thinking about it? If you can, then it doesn't matter.

You will enjoy the world when you know how to handle it well, when you become master of it. Who is the man who enjoys food? The one who eats well, chews well, digests well, and assimilates well, not the one who eats for the sake of his tongue, overloads his stomach, and then uses purgatives.

A Yogi is like a surfer who knows how to balance on his board. He welcomes even a big, rolling wave because he knows how to enjoy it without getting caught in it. A man who doesn't know how to surf will get rolled by the wave.

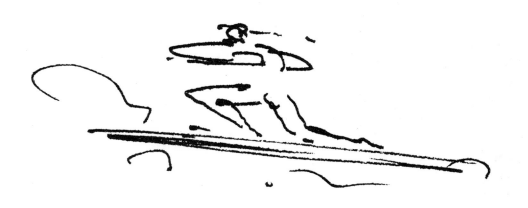

If your friends laugh at you and say, "You are just running away from the world, you are not going to enjoy anything." Tell them, "We are the people who are going to enjoy it best because we are working to bring everything under our control. We don't want to be controlled by anything. We want to be masters of our tongues and our eyes. If we want to eat, we eat. If we don't, we won't. We won't be a slave to our desires." Ask them if they can exercise their mastery like that. This is the aim of Yoga.

If you believe in something, practice it in your own life. We don't want preachers, we want people to practice. Let it take time. Nothing is achieved overnight.

Many people today want everything quickly. There is a sense of haste, of urgency. We live in an age of speed. But what is gained in speed is lost in power, and what is gained in power is lost in speed. If you gain speed by shifting into the highest gear, you can't climb a steep hill. If you want to carry a load and climb uphill, shift into low gear.

People want to get instant bliss, so they take drugs. They get high, but they lose all their power. They don't even have the power to come back and stay where they were. Many people who were in a terrible hurry and took hundreds of trips are tripping today. They trip with every step they take.

If you really want something genuine and pure, you need not go out and search for it. It's already given to you. Your peace, happiness, health, spirituality—anything you want, all these things are in you.

There is a natural way to unfold your consciousness and expand your mind. Imagine a person wanting to go from the ground floor to the top floor. If somebody puts him into a rocket and launches him, he won't land comfortably because he is not moving within his own capacity.

The same thing happens when people try to expand their consciousness with chemicals and drugs. The conscious mind is suddenly suppressed and the subconscious mind unleashed. It shakes the nerves, glands, everything.

Mind expansion should be practiced consciously, through concentration, meditation, controlling the senses, and working on the physical body with Hatha Yoga and breathing exercises. Then you will see gradual, safe progress.

Everybody wants to develop their extrasensory perception. To them I say, even with limited-sensory perception you are in a lot of trouble. Many things are purposely hidden. When you are a child, you are given only a small allowance. As you grow up, it is gradually increased.

In the same way, the divine Mother Nature within waits for your maturity. She is ready to put everything in your hands. But if you demand it prematurely, you are asking for trouble.

So instead of trying to handle God's power, let God handle you when you are ready. That should be your approach to Yoga. Refine yourself, and when you are ready, the *Kundalini* force will reveal itself and bring all powers.

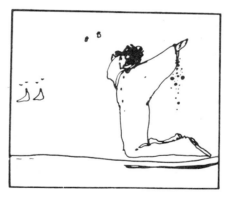

I recommend that Yoga practitioners not do any strenuous practices to arouse the Kundalini prematurely. It is there waiting for you. You don't want your fruits and vegetables to be ripened quickly with chemicals. You want a natural growth. Let your system also grow naturally. Let it be refined naturally. And then, at a certain point, you will be a fit instrument.

How does the Kundalini work? Physically, the major part of the Cosmic Consciousness in you is stored at the base of the spine. When you are ready, it gets awakened. It moves slowly up the spine toward the brain, awakening all the psychic powers located in different parts of the spine, which are called *chakras.*

Any chakra below the heart will have animalistic tendencies that pull you down. If the Kundalini rises by itself, it will pass through all these chakras. It will come to the heart right away, and then go up farther.

But if you are a glutton and do violent practices to awaken the Kundalini when your concentration is on the lower chakras, you will become more hungry. If you have sexual inclinations and that chakra opens up, you won't be able to control your sexual appetite. So it's not advisable to arouse Kundalini quickly. Let it rise up in a peaceful way when you are purified.

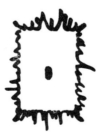

Electricity is generated by thousands of volts. We can't approach it directly, so it has to be transformed by step-down transformers. When it comes to your home, it comes as 110 volts, so that even if you get a shock, you won't be electrocuted. Suppose you say, "I want the big current. I'm a rich man and my house must have more voltage." Then you'll have bigger shocks also. God's power is like that. You have to learn how to handle it, how to protect yourself.

In the last century, there was a great saint named St. Ramalinga Swamigal who lived in South India. Nobody could photograph him, though many people tried. He was a great *siddha,* meaning he could do anything and everything. Sri Ramalingam used to present himself in various places at the same time.

One day he was sitting in his ashram talking to people. While he was talking, he suddenly pulled the turban from his head, squeezed it, and said, "Careless priest!" His followers asked for an explanation. He said, "That priest was careless. He set fire to the curtain in front of the altar." Sixty miles away, at a holy place he frequently visited, a priest had been waving a camphor light in front of the shrine. The curtain caught fire so St. Ramalingam squeezed the turban and put it out.

Such things are possible even today. But these powers are not the goal. They just come as by-products of concentration and purification and are used when there is a need, not to show off. St. Ramalingam was able to control the elements. But he made a mistake in revealing his capabilities, because even after years of preaching to people to be good, to practice meditation, to pray and trust in God, they only wanted miracles. They came thinking he would do something to them without their own effort, so they never let his words of advice change their lives.

He became disappointed and toward the very end of his life he said, "I opened my shop but people wanted unnecessary things. There were not enough people to buy the right things so I'm closing my shop and going away."

Those were his last words. He went into a room and asked his devotees to lock the door and not open it. The room had only one door. When the authorities heard of this, they said, "You can't do that! You can't lock somebody in. It's against the law."

So the officials came and ordered the room opened. The disciples refused to disobey their master's order. The officials said, "If you won't, we will." When they opened the door, there was nobody there. St. Ramalingam had just disappeared.

By controlling the prana, or life energy that is within the microcosm, you gain mastery and victory over the entire macrocosm. When you can control the prana inside you, you can control the prana outside. They are one and the same force on different levels.

Scientists work hard with the outside matter and need all kinds of technological instruments to harness it. If you have inner control, you can harness the outside matter without any instruments by your mere will. But our goal should not be that. Our goal should be to keep the mind and senses clean and to use them for the sake of humanity.

You can attain this by the sincere practice of Yoga. And when I say Yoga, I do not mean Hatha Yoga alone. Yoga means everything: asanas, pranayama, sense control, concentration, meditation, purity of mind, a dedicated life, a compassionate heart, a strong will, and forgetting one's own selfishness. All these things should be expressed in our lives. Then we will become strong, peaceful, joyful, and useful.

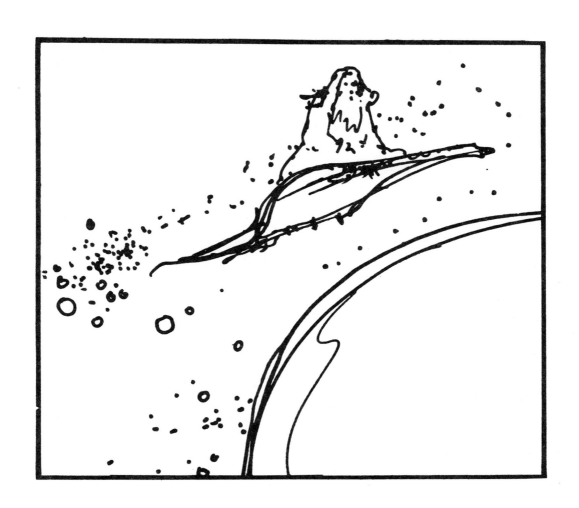

YOU ARE THE
CAUSE OF IT ALL

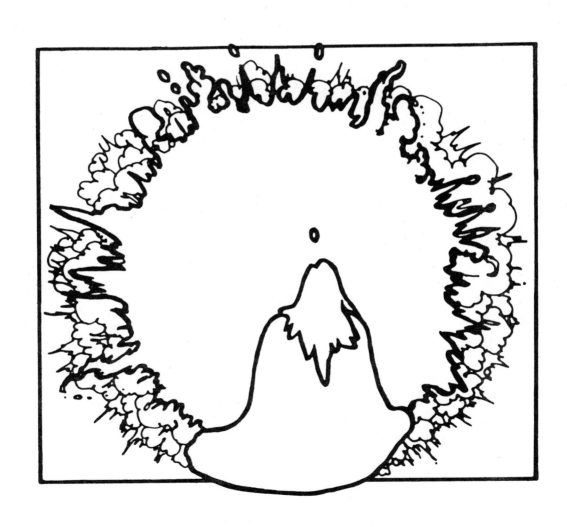

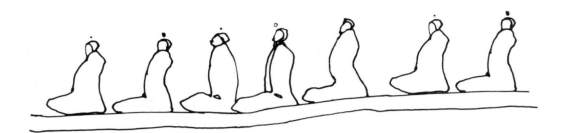

Go to Detroit and see an automobile factory. Not all cars on the assembly line are finished. In one section, you see finished cars; in another, cars 80 percent finished; in another, cars 50 percent finished; in still another, you find the spare parts and crude materials.

The world is a big factory or assembly line, constantly producing and refining people. The refined ones are not involved in the factory process. They are out in the showcase for others to see.

A man once went into a Hindu temple and stood looking at a statue. All of a sudden, he heard a soft conversation. The stone on the floor in front of the statue asked the statue, "How come all these people decorate you with nice ornaments and worship before you, but walk on me and ignore me completely?"

"You could be having the same treatment as me," replied the statue, "but you missed your opportunity. The sculptor who made me brought a big stone to his studio. When he found out the stone was too big, he broke it in half. I was one piece and you were the other. He started working on you first. He placed his chisel and gave a little tap. Immediately you shouted at him, 'Ouch! Don't touch me! How dare you hit me!'

He thought you were possessed with some devil so he put you aside and started working on me. I thought there must be some reason behind all his hits and decided to wait and see. I waited patiently and little by little, he chiseled off all the unwanted pieces. He didn't create me. A statue was always there, hidden in the stone. All he did was chisel away the unwanted pieces and my form emerged. That is the reason you are there and I am here."

Like the statue, we should understand the purpose of difficulties and pain in life. It's like surgery, painful but beneficial. A mother who gives birth to a child faces a lot of suffering. But beyond that suffering she knows she is going to have a lovely baby so she faces it and accepts it.

If the pain in our lives is properly understood, it will never frighten us. We might even welcome it, saying, "Come on, pain, help me get rid of all this dross. Refine me."

The more you heat and melt gold, the more it improves its quality. If you want to make 14-carat gold into 22-carat gold, heat it, melt it, and heat it again. Every time you do that, it loses some of its impurities and becomes refined.

When your own fineness is lost, you "re-fine" it. Whoever has done that is called a refined person. "Refinement" means you have done something to return to the fine-ness.

You were originally fine but you "de-fined" yourself: "I am an American, he is an Australian. I am young, he is old. I am black, he is white." These are all your definitions.

These definitions limit us. We have to remove our definitions and that process is called refinement. Once you get that refinement, you are one with everybody and fine again.

Often, the path seems difficult and unrewarding. When you're learning to play the piano, you hit many undesirable notes. Your neighbors complain constantly. They all wait for you to close the piano and walk away. It takes a long time to perfect your playing.

If you want to get an immediate reward, do something small. If you plant a spinach seed, you get spinach quickly. But if you want a tall tree to give fruit for years and years, you can't expect it all in one day. A guinea pig may give a dozen babies after a pregnancy of just two months, but you may have to wait as long as eighteen months for an elephant to have even one baby.

Everything worthwhile takes its own time. If you attempt perfection in one day, you are not going to achieve much of anything. This applies especially to developing the spiritual force, the willpower. Begin with little things, daily, and one day you will be doing things that months back you would have thought were impossible. That is the way you develop your will.

Apply your will to a thing that is possible for you to do.

Don't try a thing that is very difficult or beyond your capacity. Say, for example, you are a person who takes three spoons of sugar in every cup of tea. Say, "All right, from morning to evening, I will take only two spoons." Tomorrow you say, "Instead of taking ten cups of tea I will take five," or "Instead of ten cigarettes, I will only smoke seven."

Little by little you develop your will. It's something like teaching a baby to walk, one small step at a time. The baby tries, falls, gets up, and you say, "You are really great! Now, come on, take another bigger step!" That is the way you teach. The mind is so weak and childish you have to train it slowly.

If you can do what you have decided to do, without any excuse, postponement, laziness, or delay, you have applied your will. You want to do something and you do it. And even wanting to do something should have a weight to it. Some people say, "Well, I will see, I'll try . . ." They say, "I will try," as if they have no confidence even in their trying. Such people cannot apply their will.

Instead, if they say, "I will try that and somehow will achieve it," the very affirmation, the very beginning has strength. When you think, "I seem to be able to do anything I want," then you really are capable of doing anything and everything you want. You have faith in your own Self and self-confidence.

Always remember your goal. If you understand the goal and dedicate yourself to achieving it, you won't get disheartened by failure. The very interest in achieving the goal will take you to it.

Failure is natural. We should not get disheartened by failure. Nobody has ever achieved something great without failing. Ask yourself why you failed and learn something. Every failure must be a stepping-stone for your further success. Use all the failures as stepping-stones, one after another; then they are helpful experiences.

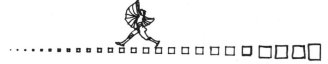

You can't run away from problems. You will face the same problems wherever you go. They are teachers. The mathematics professor gives you problems. When you find solutions, he promotes you. Nature functions the same way. If you run away from problems and transfer into another school, a teacher there will give you the same problems until you solve them. That is life.

It is only by mistakes that we learn. Only by falling do we learn to walk. It is difficult to visualize a world without problems. Can you have an examination hall without question papers? Each question is a problem to you. However much you scratch your head, you have to find a solution. If you find one, you pass.

Problems help us develop our inner resources. It is through problems that we learn. We should never expect a smooth, problem-free world. In such a world there would be no learning or growing.

Take a seed, for example. If the seed is left on a plate, it will just remain there. It won't grow. If you dig a hole and bury it, the seed faces a problem: "How can I get sunlight? I am buried. I can't sleep here. I must get out." And in its effort to escape, the seed reveals the beautiful tree within. If you say, "I don't want to create problems for the seed, let me leave it on the plate," the seed will remain a seed. It won't get an opportunity to express itself and grow. That is the way we should understand problems. Every problem is there to help you bring forth your own capabilities.

Other people who are able to solve problems can guide you by saying, "This is the way we solved our problems. Try it." Others can't solve your problems, but they can tell you how they solved theirs. That's why you don't go to a person who has a lot of unsolved problems to help you solve your own.

We act as if problems came from outside. We try to blame someone else and say, "He caused the problem. She caused the problem. This or that caused the problem." The nature of the human mind is to blame somebody or something.

Imagine someone walking along the road. All of a sudden, he tumbles down and gets hurt. If you ask him what happened, he says, "A stone tripped me." We never think in terms of what we did to cause a problem. We must learn to turn inward to find out the cause.

You are your own problem, your own friend, and your own enemy. In other words, if your mind is a good friend to you, you will see only friends everywhere. But if your own mind acts like a traitor, you will find few friends. So make your mind your friend. Let it not color your vision. Let it not prejudice your thinking. It can be a beautiful instrument with which you can understand things well.

Truly speaking, there is neither good nor bad in the world outside. Everything is neutral. Take an electric outlet, for example. Is it good or bad? You say, "Oh, it is very good. When I plug in a lamp, I get light. When I plug in a radio, I get music."

All of a sudden somebody jumps up and says, "No. Electricity is very dangerous. The other day I plugged my finger into an electrical outlet and got a terrible shock!" To him, electricity is terrible.

The moment we hear the word *poison* we are frightened. But certain medicines are made from poison. Poison can be nectar if you know how to use it.

If you go and lean against a wall, it helps you. If you bump your head against it, it hurts you. The wall has no desire to create a bump on your head or to help you support yourself. You go to it and get the reward or punishment according to your approach.

The Lord has no special interest in rewarding you or punishing you. You are the lord of your own punishment or reward. All the Lord does is to see that you get a proper reaction to your action. If you put your finger in the fire, it will burn. God is not going to force you to put your finger into the fire. It's up to you. God simply sees that if you sow an apple seed, an apple tree comes up, not a rosebush.

What you sow, you reap. That is the Lord's way. That's why you don't need to praise the Lord for happiness or blame the Lord for unhappiness. You are the cause of it all.

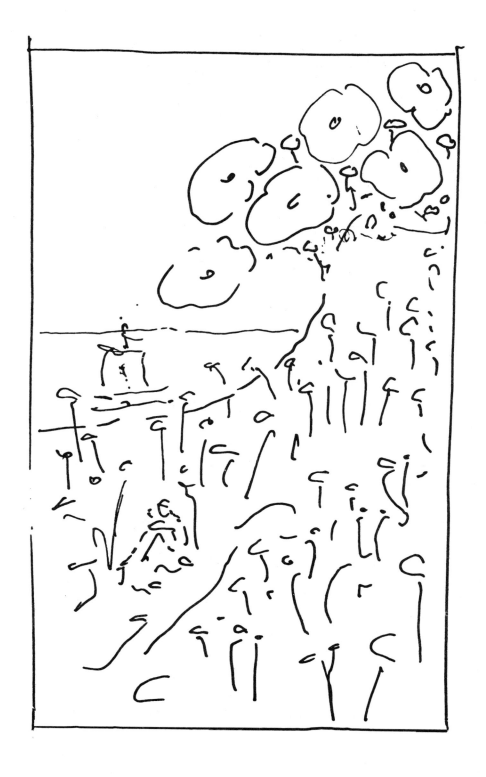

MIND

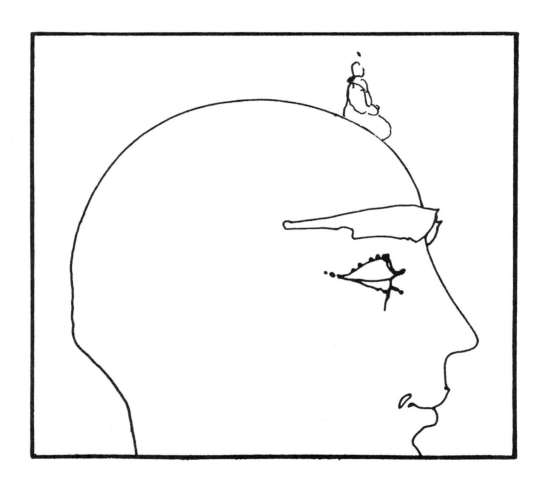

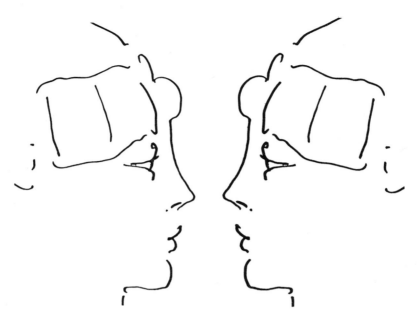

Have you ever seen your own face? No. What you see in a mirror is not your face. It's a reflection. If, to your great surprise, your face looks horrible and distorted in the mirror, do you jump up and run to the hospital? No, you get another mirror.

You know that the problem is with the mirror and not your face. A distorted mirror will make your face appear distorted. To see your face as it really is, you need a clean, straight mirror.

In a glass mirror, you can see your face. But what is the mirror with which you can see your True Self? The mind. The mind is the mirror of the Self. Your True Self is never ugly, never restless, never dirty. It is the image of God and God is never unhappy. If the mind is clean and straight, you see a true picture of yourself; you see yourself as peaceful and happy. But when the mind becomes dirty or restless, you see a horrible reflection of your Self and think *you* yourself are horrible.

84

When people take themselves to be their disturbed minds, they want to escape that horrible reflection immediately. Some buy tranquilizers, some drink, and some smoke grass. We have instant coffee and instant tea, why not instant tranquility and bliss?

We want our bodies to be organic and try to eat organic foods. Shouldn't our minds be organic also? Why use chemicals? Whether it is a pill, grass, a fix, whatever, the tranquility it brings is chemically produced. Bliss is natural. You don't need to get or create bliss, you are bliss.

You don't have to do anything to keep the mind calm. It's like a bowl of water. Should you do anything to keep the water peaceful? Just leave it alone. *Let it be.* That's the song you sing. The very same thing has been said in all religions. Let it be. So be it. Amen. You don't need to become anything. All you have to do is to be.

People often ask me, "What religion are you? You talk about the Bible, Koran, Torah. Are you a Hindu?" I say, "I am not a Catholic, a Buddhist, or a Hindu, but an Undo. My religion is Undoism. We have done enough damage. We have to stop doing any more and simply undo the damage we have already done."

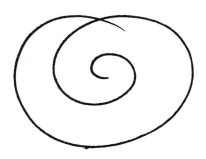

If I ask the question, "Who are you?" and record all the answers I get, the list would read something like, "I am a man; I am a woman; I am black; I am white; I am slim; I am fat; I am a doctor; I am a philosopher."

If you write all these answers one below the other, take a long cardboard and cover the first two words *I am,* you see *man, woman, black, white, slim, fat, doctor, philosopher.* If you move the cardboard and cover the other half, you see, *I am, I am, I am, I am.*

We all agree on the first half and disagree on the second. I am means *I am.* Not that I was or I will be. I am, right now, in the present.

Anything you call "mine" is not you. "My house" is not me, "my hand" is not me. "My body" is not me then, either. If it is me, how can I say "my body"? When we identify ourselves as the mind or the body, we say things like, "I was happy. Now I am depressed."

When you are depressed or excited, pull back and ask, "Who is depressed? Who is excited? Me? Certainly not. It must be my mind." The minute you separate yourself from your mind, it's as if a main switch has been turned off and the agony is gone. You become the person who is witnessing things. You don't need to get lost in your ups and downs.

What is a depression? It's part of a wave. A wave is one-half depression and one-half crest. If you want to cause a wave on a tranquil sheet of water, just throw something in. When something falls in, it creates a depression first. Adjoining the depression, a crest of water is formed. The crest is your effort to fulfill the depression. The cause of depression is a desire, or a want, that has fallen into your mind.

There is nothing wrong in your getting exposed to things. Just don't want them for yourself. Don't go and develop or brood over them. It's something like exposing movie film. If you take the film out of the camera before it gets developed and hold it up to a light, all the images will be erased.

Open up your reel of film in the light of God. Open your heart, don't keep it a dark chamber. You constantly take pictures. You have many lenses and microphones, so it's a touching, smelling, stereo, 3-D movie. At the end of the day open up your camera. Say, "These are all the shots I exposed today. It's all for You, not for me." You expose everything and He disposes of it, keeping your film clean.

And what is film? It's a plain sheet coated with a sensitive chemical, like silver nitrate. Once the chemical is applied, the film cannot be exposed to light. The treated film is then placed in a dark box that we call the camera. Every time you open the lens, light enters and the camera takes a picture. The length of the exposure depends on the sensitivity of the coating. The sensitivity is measured in ASA numbers. *Asa* in Sanskrit means desire.

After you develop the exposed film, you have to put it in the fixing bath. Once you fix it, you can't easily erase it. The fixed film is put on the projector. Whatever has been exposed, developed, and fixed is seen on the screen. The image appears on the screen but never affects the screen. In the same way, the film never affects the inner bulb but just throws its shadows onto the screen.

And where does all this happen? In a dark hall. If anyone wants to see the picture more clearly and points a flashlight at the screen, he won't see anything there. From the minute the film becomes sensitive, all the way up to projection, everything happens in darkness. Darkness means ignorance. That's why we say, "Lord, please lead me from this darkness to the light. I have had enough exposures, enough developments, enough fixations, and enough projections."

You are the projector and your soul is the light. The only time the screen is clear is when there is a clear film between it and the light. And what is that film? Your own mind. Originally, the mind is as clean as that plain, uncoated film. But then, by some trick of Nature or God, it gets coated with one sensitive coat of asa. What is the first coat of asa? "I." The bigger the "I," the greater the sensitivity. That's why egoistic people are more sensitive.

An open-minded person lets light into his camera. Then things come in but don't get fixed. They don't leave any trace, so he's not affected by anything. If you don't allow any light in, and think, "Ah, what a pretty thing I saw today, somehow I must get it," you have developed and fixed the depression caused by a want falling into your mind. It becomes a fixation and you run around to fulfill it.

So you fulfill it by your effort. Once the effort brings fulfillment, what do you get? You get back your normal tranquility. Not that you get anything new. Before the want, you had peace. When the desire fell in you had a depression. To fulfill the depression, you applied some energy and then you returned to your original state of peace.

But, unfortunately, you say, "I got peace, I *got* happiness." You forget why you got depressed in the first place. All you know is, "I got it, I am happy. To stay happy, I must get more." And the minute you say, "To be happy, I must get more," that is another desire, which makes another depression, and it goes on forever.

So the best approach is to know the cause of depression, to know what kind of desires cause depression. There are desires that will never cause depression, desires not based on your own selfish aims or personal benefit. Anything impersonal or unselfish will never create a depression in your mind, because you are doing it for others. You do it within your capacity and don't get depressed if you cannot do it.

Imagine you are walking by the ocean. All of a sudden you see somebody fall in. Unfortunately you don't know how to swim. Will you jump in? No. You will shout for help, but if you can't get any help, you won't get depressed. You will have done all that you could.

But if that somebody is your friend or brother, seeing him drowning upsets you. Because of that attachment you might even lose the capacity to shout for help. That is the difference between help without any personal relationship and help with some sort of personal attachment.

Be compassionate, but don't mistake compassion for depression. Be sympathetic, but don't lose your peace.

In realizing the Self you begin to understand that you are never the doer and never the enjoyer. It is the mind that does and enjoys everything. Once that realization happens, the mind becomes a beautiful instrument, never a selfish one. The minute you realize the Self, you are never worried because you know that you have never done anything.

Even if the mind undergoes certain sufferings, you can stand back and say, "Well, you did all the mischief, now purge it out." It's like a mother giving a strong purgative to her naughty child who ate too much candy. The child really undergoes pain and the mother says, "What can I do? I am just purging out all the poison. You ate everything. I told you not to. If you had not done it, you would not have to go through this."

You can advise the mind like that. "You are so selfish, you ate everything. You didn't even want to share with your brothers and sisters. So, at least in the future, remember not to go near the refrigerator." Pleasure and pain belong to the mind and not to you. Think you are unhappy and you are unhappy. Think you are happy and you are happy.

Several people were walking along the road early in the morning when they saw a man lying along by the side. The first one who saw him said, "He must have spent the whole night in the gambling dens, couldn't reach home, and fell asleep. Gamblers are always like that. They don't reach home safely."

The next person said, "Poor man. He must really be sick," and then walked away.

The third person said, "Humph! Dirty bum! You don't know how to hold your liquor. Someone probably gave you some free whiskey."

The fourth man said, "To a saint, nothing matters. He is probably above this physical consciousness. Let me not disturb him." He bowed and walked away.

We don't know who was right. All four saw the same person. But each saw him differently because each projected something of himself. The world is nothing but your projection. If there is hell in your mind, you see hell everywhere. If there is heaven in your mind, you see heaven everywhere. Correct your vision and you will see the Truth. Everything begins in the mind. If you want to see clearly, you need clear vision. Pollution begins with the mind, and then extends to the air and the earth. We project our minds onto the world.

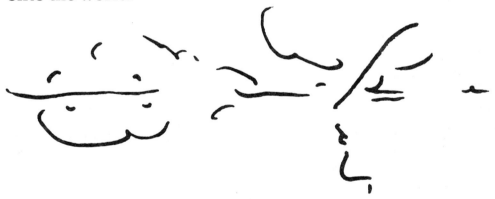

The mind is constantly being tossed about by the three qualities or, in Sanskrit, the three *gunas*: *sattwa, rajas,* and *tamas.* Sattwa is tranquility, rajas is dynamic activity, and tamas is inertness. Whenever you feel dull, lazy, or drowsy, the tamasic quality of the mind is predominant. But sometimes you can't sit quietly. You are restless. At that moment the mind is rajasic, so use the time to get things done. Finally, there are times you get into an in-between, very balanced state. You feel like doing, but not overdoing. You are neither dull nor excited. This is the sattwic state.

These changes happen without your wanting them to. That is the proof that the mind is being tossed about by the three gunas. Sometimes, when there is wind, the flame flickers. When there is no wind, the flame is steady. So when the sattwa, rajas, and tamas winds come, the mind gets caught in them.

But you can strengthen the mind. You can turn an ordinary flickering lamp into a hurricane lamp. If there's no shelter, if it's not well-protected, you have to keep a lamp indoors; you can't even open the windows. The minute you open them, the flame will blow out.

But if you shelter the flame, it can face even a hurricane. It's the same flame, but well protected. The mind is like that. You can build up strength of mind so that it can face all situations.

When you have a clean mind, you know who you are. You realize your Self. Your vision becomes spiritual. Until then, you see only through your physical or mental eye. When you see with your physical eye, you see very little. With the mental eye, you can see much more. But with the spiritual eye, you see the Truth.

No thought is new. It is all already there. There is no past, present, or future. Everything is the present, right here and now, but you see only a part of it, which becomes your present. If you make your vision more wide-angled, you see more.

Man is created by thought. What a man thinks, he becomes. Man sows a thought and reaps an action, sows an action and reaps a habit, sows a habit and reaps a destiny. Man has made his destiny by his thinking. By right thinking, he can become the master of his destiny instead of a slave to it. The greatest victory you can win is over your own mind.

God plus mind is man. Man minus mind is God.

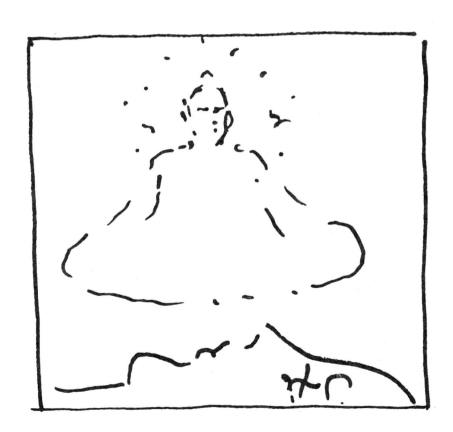

MEDITATION

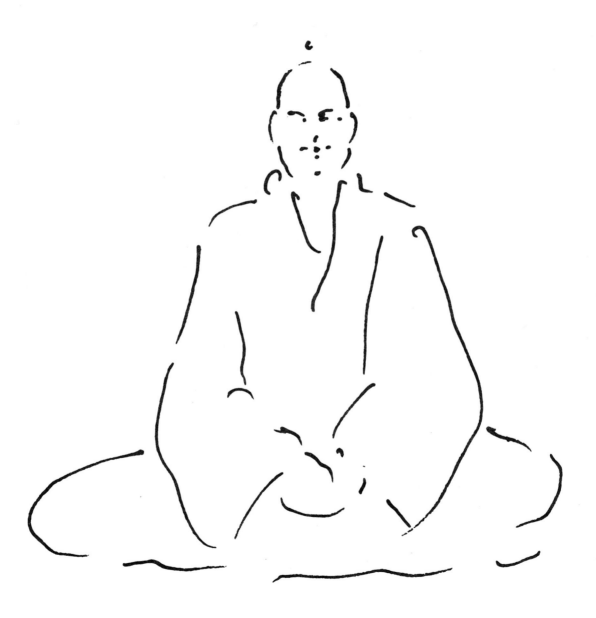

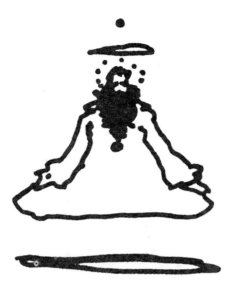

Yoga means getting yourself one-pointed and training your mind to do one thing at a time. Work while you work, play while you play. Eat while you eat, and sleep while you sleep.

We all have this capacity. But because we don't apply our entire mind and focus all its energies one hundred percent on the work at hand, we don't penetrate into the depth of it and attain what should be attained. The secret of success is to gather your mind. Once you gather the mind totally to one point, it becomes the greatest power on earth.

You can't thread a needle if the end of the thread isn't sharp enough. It's the same with the mind. All the ideas and all the thought forms must be concentrated on one thing; then they gain strength. If you detonate a bullet outside a gun, it explodes. But if you detonate it in a gun barrel, it has to take the path of the barrel. It runs through the barrel and builds up momentum until it penetrates the target.

Concentration means focusing all the thoughts to a center. Unless the sun's rays are focused, they won't bring heat. Unless the flowing river is dammed up and focused into a tube, you won't get hydroelectricity. Unless gasoline passes from the tank into the carburetor and is focused onto the exact point in the compression chamber, the engine won't deliver its power.

Like the point of a drill, our mind can penetrate into anything to know its secret. If you gather all the thought forms, collect them together, and concentrate them on one idea or object, they penetrate, reveal, and arrive at the inner secret of that idea. That is what inventors do. Their minds are focused. Their concentration is so deep that nature reveals its secrets to them.

With that control and focus you can gain anything you want in this world. Nothing is impossible for a one-pointed mind. You will always enjoy success and never complain of failure because your actions will be perfect and your mind will be at peace. This is the goal of Yoga—not just to stand on your head for ten minutes or hold your breath for a minute or two. Anybody can do that.

But even mental control is not enough. You can control the mind, focus it, and discover all of nature's secrets. But then you must know how to handle and make use of them. You need the proper understanding to use them properly, a pure mind, a broad mind, and a desireless mind. That means a selfless mind.

Otherwise, you will try to possess all the secrets you discover for yourself. That's why, even today, with all our scientific inventions, we are not peaceful or happy. We are anxious and fearful, because nature's secrets are controlled by the wrong minds. In the wrong hands, they disturb and frighten the world.

Every day we try to learn more and more—to discover things. The world is in chaos because many secrets and great energies have been unearthed. They have been let loose and man finds it difficult to control them.

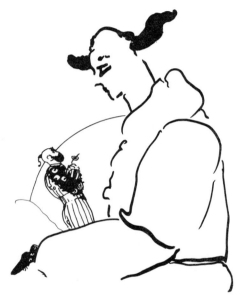

Once a man wanted to perform extraordinary feats, so he went into the forest and approached a sorcerer. The sorcerer told him, "I can give you a big demon who will do everything for you. But be careful. You must always be able to give him work. If you don't, he will devour you." The man said, "There is a lot to do in this world. Don't worry, I can easily find work for ten demons."

So the sorcerer gave him the spell with which he could summon the demon. At the proper time, the demon appeared and asked, "My Master, why did you call me? I have come, give me some work." The man immediately said, "I want a huge palace with many rooms. Build one and fill it with beautiful furnishings from around the world."

He thought that building such a big palace and furnishing it would take a while so he decided to go to sleep until the demon was finished. He was about to lie down when the demon appeared and said, "Master, your palace is ready." And there it was, a huge palace, fully furnished.

The man thought for a second and said, "I must have a hundred servants to keep everything in order." "Yes, Master," said the demon, snapping his fingers, "the servants are already there, taking care of everything." "I need some cars," said the man. "Beautiful cars, Master, Rolls-Royces and Cadillacs, with drivers and a private filling station. All is ready." "I am hungry," said the man. "A gourmet meal, with maids to serve it, is waiting in the dining room," replied the demon.

The man was a little puzzled. "What's going on here?" he asked. "The minute I ask for something, you make it appear. It doesn't even take a second." "Don't hesitate," said the demon. "Give me some work. I can't be without work. Give me something to do!"

The man didn't quite know what to say because the demon didn't ever give him time to think about what he wanted done next. He tried his best to give work to the demon, but everything got done immediately. Then the demon said, "Either give me more work or I'll devour you."

The man ran back to the sorcerer but the sorcerer wasn't there. Sitting nearby was a holy man. He fell at the holy man's feet saying, "A demon is after me. If I don't give him something to do, he will devour me, and I've run out of things for him to do! Can you help me, please?"

"Yes, my son," said the saint. He plucked one of his very curly hairs and gave it to the man, saying, "Bring this to the demon and ask him to keep it straight." The man returned and ordered the demon to perform this new task. The demon held the bottom of the hair in one hand, slowly pulled it up straight with the other, and then let it go. It sprang right back and curled up. Again he tried, and again it sprang back.

"Have you finished straightening it?" asked the man.
"No, I'm still trying," replied the demon.
"Well," said the man, "finish quickly because I have some other work for you to do!"

The demon's work was now to straighten the hair. Whenever the man needed other work done, he called the demon, who would leave the hair temporarily, do the new work in a second, and then return to his task. From then on, the demon always had something to do and was under control.

Every one of us has been given a demon. It resides within us and is our own mind. It is restless. It always wants to do something. It induces us to do this and that. Day and night the mind extracts work because it has no other work to do. Like a rudderless, anchorless boat tossed in the ocean by a terrible wind, the restless mind runs here and there and doesn't want to keep quiet. If you want to put it in one place where it won't disturb you, give it a curly hair.

That curly hair is your mantram. Give it to your mind and say, "Repeat this and don't bother me. Don't push me here and there. Do this work, and when I want your full attention for something, you can leave it and come to me." Then the mind is calmed and under control.

Repetition of a mantram is the simplest and best practice for concentration. It can be practiced by everybody, without any restrictions. You don't need any special time, you don't need to carry things around, because it is always with you. You can repeat your mantram in the middle of work, when you cook, and when you eat.

When the mind is made to focus on one point and that one-pointedness is achieved continuously, you call that meditation. When that meditation on the mantram is well developed, undesirable thoughts will become weaker and stop troubling you. It's something like going into a field of weeds and planting a powerful seed that will bring forth a big tree. When that seed grows into a tree, it will suck away all the nourishment for itself and, automatically, the weeds will die. Develop one powerful thought which will not bind you, which will make you more universal and selfless, and the worldly thoughts will slowly become weaker.

Ultimately, you have to free your mind from everything. By giving you a mantram, we are only giving you something that will not bother you later on. When you squeeze fresh grease into your car's engine, the old grease is automatically forced out. By repeating the mantram you are putting fresh grease in your mind and forcing out all the old grease. Then everything will run smoothly.

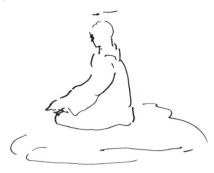

We should prepare for meditation as we prepare for sleep. We don't just throw ourselves into bed. We change our dress, perhaps have a warm bath, and, if necessary, a soothing, warm beverage to drink.

One has to sit in a comfortable position for meditation, either cross-legged on the floor, or in a comfortable but not easy chair. If it is an easy chair, you will become lazy. The chair should be fairly comfortable but, at the same time, you should not slouch back. To stay alert, always keep the spine erect because your spiritual force ascends through it and the ladder must be straight.

Don't worry about your legs. You can even stretch them out for a change, if necessary. It doesn't matter. But don't keep changing position. You may say, "I'm only a beginner. How can I remain in one posture?" That thinking itself will make it more difficult.

Look at your legs and say, "I have been listening to you and obeying you all these years. Now you must obey me. I am going to put you in this position. Make no complaints. Even if you complain, I am not going to listen to you. I know you won't break."

Be very strict and positive about it. Your own firmness will be understood and accepted by your legs. Don't think they are ignorant or inert. Every cell knows what you are thinking and what you are going to do. With all that, if it really becomes painful, there's no point in meditating on the pain so move a little bit. That will satisfy the body and let it think it has won a victory. But your meditation will be better if you sit still with your spine erect.

The next thing is to regulate the breathing, for the mind and the breath always go together. When the mind gets agitated, you can see the breath getting agitated. When the mind is peaceful and calm, the breath flows calmly and rhythmically. Relax and take a few slow, deep breaths, with the entire mind watching the breath. Follow the breath and let it be deep. Then, slowly allow the breath to take its own course while continuing to observe it.

After watching the breath, sit and watch your thoughts. Be a separate entity from your mind. See all that's happening in your mind. Follow the mind's natural flow. But remember that watching and analyzing the thoughts are two different things. When you judge the thoughts, you are not watching them, you are analyzing. A judge in court is not a witness. A judge analyzes who is right and who is wrong. But a witness just says what he saw.

People go to the cinema to watch and enjoy the movie, to be witnesses. But sometimes they forget that and start judging, "Look at that. The cameraman made a mistake!" They become critics, and when you are a critic you don't enjoy the film. The minute you find a criticism, your mind stays on that and you miss many other points you might otherwise appreciate.

Being a real witness means you watch everything and remain unaffected. When the hero makes love to the heroine, it's beautiful. When the villain snatches her, it's also beautiful. The mind is a movie theater. In meditation you may see divine things and then horrible pictures. Neither be attracted nor frightened by them. They're just the different impressions previously recorded by your mind. Learn to watch it all. Let the film keep rolling.

Before long, you will see the mind getting tired and slowly coming back to rest in one place. That is your opportunity to bring it to one point.

Slowly begin repeating a chosen mantram or prayer, whatever it may be. It can be "Hari Om, Hari Om, Hari Hari Hari Om," "Om Shanthi, Om Shanthi," "Amen Jesus, Amen Jesus," "Adonai Adonai," or "Shalom," according to your faith. Put your entire mental awareness on the repetition of your mantram and then, after a while, let the breath repeat it while you simply sit and watch. Choose anything that pleases you, but remember that when you meditate on higher ideas and divine spiritual qualities, you will receive them. And stick to one thing; don't keep changing.

There are many bridges and tunnels leading into Manhattan. Pick the one that's the most convenient, take it into Manhattan, and then do what you came to Manhattan to do. Later, if you have some extra time and feel like playing, you can experiment with some of the other approaches.

If you have a mantram given to you by a teacher or organization, you can continue with it. Mantrams are more or less the same. It is your faith that is important. You should repeat your mantram with full faith. If you do it with half a heart, it won't bring good results. But if you see some results and are growing, continue.

During meditation, it's natural for the mind to wander here and there but gently bring it back again and again to your mantram. It might go to a supermarket or to a cinema, but it will know that you are watching, and return. Imagine you have a pet dog at home and you never tie it up. It runs around everywhere. One day an elderly visitor whom you respect comes to your home. You don't want your dog to annoy him, so you tie it up in another room.

And then the trouble begins! Before, the dog ran around and you probably didn't even know it was there. But the minute you tie it up, it starts barking and jumping and scratching at everything. It's the same with the mind. When you begin to control it, naturally it rebels.

Don't give up. Know that you are in a circus ring. You have wild animals inside your mind, cunning foxes, tigers, and cobras. Keep the whip and snap it loudly. Use all your tactics because the mind won't easily be tamed. Once you bring it under your control, you are the master. Unless you master your own body and mind, you cannot master anything else.

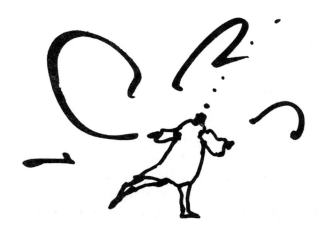

Each time the mind evades you, runs here and there, and you bring it back, that is called concentration. Concentration is trying to fix the mind on one thing. Meditation is when you have tried and are successful.

Many people think meditation means making the mind vacant. You can never make the mind vacant. The mind can become vacant but you can never make it so. When the very thought that you are trying to sleep is forgotten, you are sleeping. In the same way, when your mind is totally focused on your object of concentration, then that one thought also is dropped and the mind becomes naturally vacant.

Many people get discouraged with meditation because they expect something to happen immediately. They wait for visions or things that they read about in books. The moment they close their eyes they feel, "This must happen, that must happen because it happens to everyone else." They create a barrier, become tense, and the very tension disturbs their meditation.

Suppose you sow a seed, pour a little water on it, and then dig it up. If you don't see a root, you close the hole, pour on a little more water, and go away. The following day, you come and dig it up again to see whether it has grown. It will never grow that way. Just pour the water and leave it. The root will come in time. Our very haste in wanting the root and the fruit disturbs the seed.

In meditation, the thoughts in the subconscious mind come to the surface. They run around, try to escape, and you may see them as lights or hear them as sounds. You are beginning to recognize inner impressions. When you concentrate, you are trying to still the conscious mind. When you still the conscious mind, you get into the subconscious, which is filled with millions and millions of thought forms.

Be patient and continue repeating your mantram. It's like trying to clean a rug. A lot of dust will come up, so you need a powerful vacuum. Real enlightenment means quieting and then transcending both the conscious and subconscious mind and recognizing, or realizing, your own peace, joy, and eternal bliss. And that is Yoga. That is Christhood and Buddhahood. You are freed from turmoil. You become naked and clean. Nirvana means "nakedness." Your soul is not colored or covered by anything.

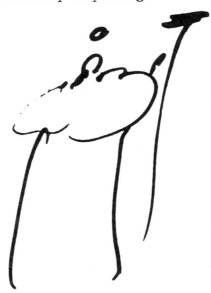

Ultimately, meditation should be continuous, not just one day a week or fifteen minutes in the morning and evening. The meditation process can continue even in your eating, breathing, working, in whatever you do. If you hold the rudder for only ten minutes and then let the wind toss the boat any way it wants, you won't reach the shore.

Say you set your boat on a particular course of 180 degrees. You may say, "I'm just a few degrees off, it doesn't matter." But where will you end up? Certainly not where you wanted to go. That's why constant attention and awareness are necessary. Somebody must hold the wheel and watch the compass. If by any chance you make a mistake and get caught by a wind, then you must correct your course. On a ship or a plane, without that course correction, you can never reach your destination. If you start in New York, wanting to go to Los Angeles, you will probably end up in Miami.

Where there is movement, there must be direction. Without direction, movement is wasted. We call that direction discipline. Imagine what would happen if cars were not disciplined on a highway! The car is directed by its steering, and the person who does the steering is directed by the goal of reaching a certain place. Movement is directed toward taking you where you want to go.

The same with the mind. If a man's mind moves without direction, we call him an aimless wanderer. His life is vague, so he is called a "vague-a-bond." We should have goals and direction. Some people call me for an appointment, come to see me, then don't know what to say. Before you do something, before you act, there should be a purpose. Know first and then act. We must be conscious of every thought and every action. Nothing should happen without our knowledge.

Not knowing does not give you a license to do the wrong things. When you drive the wrong way in one-way traffic and get a ticket or have an accident, you can't give ignorance as an excuse. You will still get the ticket or have the accident.

Anything done in a haphazard way is un-Yogic. Orderliness and beauty in your work is Yogic. When you write something, write it neatly. When you iron something, iron it in the proper way. The minute you get up, the bed should be made. The minute you change a dress, take the old dress and put it in the proper place. Don't just throw things here and there. Put everything in its place.

Sometimes people take hours looking through a drawer for an old letter. They pull out all the other letters and mix everything up. But if you keep things orderly, you can open the drawer, put your hand on the particular letter, and take it out without even seeing it.

In nature, everything is orderly. There is beauty in everything. Nothing is thrown haphazardly into this world. Beauty and order is the natural way. We should try to live with nature without disturbing its order.

In the name of Yoga, let us create a new feeling. Everything must be spotless and clean. We have to learn discipline. Take even a small flower in the garden and see how well arranged the petals are, how organized, symmetrical, and beautiful it is. Or look at the order and structure of a crystal. Discipline is what you see in nature. Everything has its place.

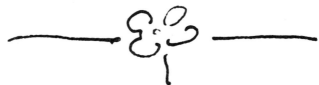

We can train our mind like that. Even in Hatha Yoga there is an orderliness and grace. By moving the body in a graceful, smooth way, the mind follows and there is no restlessness.

Don't think that meditation alone can control the mind. Constantly keep your mind on the goal of regularity and discipline. Discipline makes your mind stronger and one-pointed. It should not make you a slave. It should ultimately help you make your mind your slave. You are the master. Your mind should obey you.

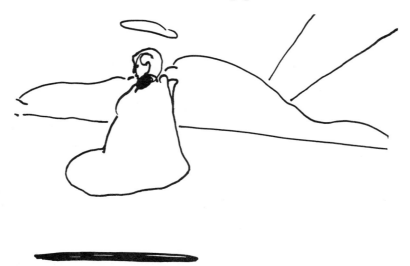

When spiritual vibrations are passed to you through a mantram or sound formula, it is called initiation. Of course, you can just pick out any mantram from a book and start repeating it. But the function of initiation by a qualified person is like the function of yogurt culture dropped into a well-prepared pot of milk.

As you know, cold milk cannot be converted into yogurt. You must first boil it well and then cool it down to the proper temperature. Then drop in a little of yesterday's yogurt as the culture. Allow the culture to work. Take the pot and put it somewhere overnight. In the morning, you will see the milk has become steady and solid. If you then want butter, which is even more solid, churn it. Heat will be produced and the fat, or butter, separates and floats.

If you pour the original milk into water, the two immediately mix together. But if you throw a ball of butter into the same water, it will float. In the same way, our minds in the beginning are like liquid. And very often they are cold. So to get spiritual experience, or to find the essence of the mind, we have to boil it first. When your mind is boiling, you become a seeker asking, "Where can I go? Who can put a little culture into me?"

When the teacher knows you are boiled enough, he cools you off a little. He doesn't say, "Come here. Let me put a little culture into you." First he helps you settle your mind by making you understand a little of how you should be living. Then he gives a little "culture" by passing some of his vibration to you through a mantram and a touch. You get today's culture from yesterday's culture and yesterday's culture was made from the day before yesterday's culture, and so on. So there is a tradition.

By repeating the mantram that's given to you, you develop the culture and the whole mind settles. With the mind steady, like yogurt, you will be able to inquire deeply into your essence and churn it out. When you are well churned, your true nature, the *Atman* or the butter, comes out. Then, if you throw yourself into this ocean of illusion, you will never drown. You will be in the world, but you won't be of the world. You become like a boat. A boat can carry people from shore to shore. You can be in the world without the world affecting you.

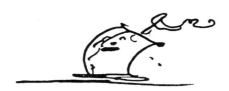

Receiving mantra initiation is like having a beautiful seed planted within you. The person who does the planting won't be able to run behind you to water and fertilize and weed it. That is your duty. Keep on watering, see that the seed gets enough nourishment, and that no wild weeds grow up.

Anything that disturbs your pure life is a weed, and it will slowly disturb the growth and take away the nourishment that you give to this seed.

The seed is powerful: even if you don't supply water and fertilizer, it will still be there. It won't die but neither will it grow. Take good care of it and it will grow and bring forth beautiful fruit.

Constant remembering and repetition is like watering. And your good associations with people who have a similar interest in life are like nourishment. Take good care of your associations, your study, your reading, your seeing, and your eating.

If you want a very simple practice, mantra meditation is the one. All other practices need a certain time, place, or equipment. You can't do Hatha Yoga when you are flying in a plane, when you are cooking, when you are on the toilet, or in the office. If you sit in the office and start doing breathing exercises, people may even get scared. But if you do your mantram, no one need know what you are doing. You can do it on the subway or in the bathtub; nothing can prevent you from remembering your mantram.

Many people say we are moving into the Aquarian Age, an era of expanded consciousness, but the one we seem to be living in now is called *Kali Yuga,* the Iron Age. It is very crude, very rough, a dull and dark age. In the Kali Yuga it is very difficult to do strenuous and difficult practices, but now especially, mantra practice is very easy and powerful. So keep it in your mind always.

Don't allow your mantram to sit there unused. It's something very precious. That's why you seldom hear me talking about mantra initiation or inviting people to it. I wait for people to find out about it and really want it. What I am giving is something very precious which should be earned and appreciated. If you do not have the interest, there's no need to give it to you. I'm not interested in making more disciples. Even if I have only ten, they should be gems. I could have truckloads of granite stones and pebbles, but what would be the use?

So let the holy vibration of your mantram develop in your heart, in your soul, in your body, and create a beautiful vibration and atmosphere around you. Then you can find that peace and joy within and make others feel the same peace when they are around you. You will be walking, living peace machines. We will be life partners. Let us go together, walk together, and pray together.

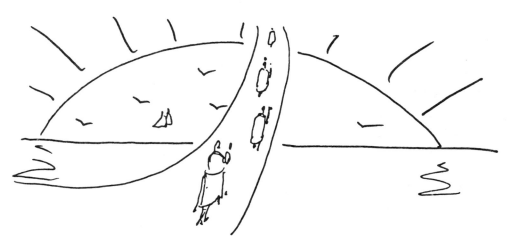

PRAYER

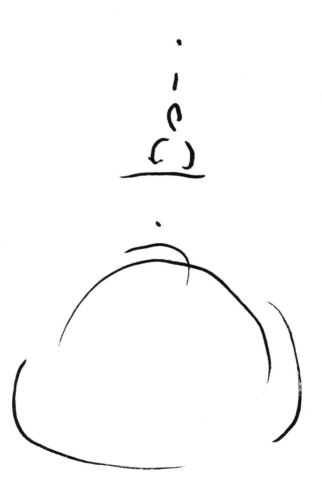

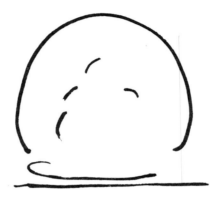

I once visited a home where there was a young baby. I was talking to the family and the mother was busy somewhere in the kitchen. The baby was playing with its toys. After a while, the baby cried a little and started putting things in its mouth, thinking that by sucking on them, it might get some milk to satisfy its hunger. A little crying, a little trying, again a little crying; this went on for a while. When it had sucked everything and not found any milk, it cried some more.

Then the mother came with a rubber pacifier. The baby started sucking the pacifier and stopped crying. But very soon it found out that milk wasn't coming even from the pacifier. Then it started kicking everything and really crying. This time the cry was completely different. And now the mother knew that the crying was real and came running to take the baby and feed it.

That taught me a very good lesson. I used to meditate and pray a little, but my mind was on the market and the cinema. I used to go to the Himalayas, sit in front of the Ganges, close my eyes, and start meditating, but I would be meditating on the cinemas of New Delhi. I would be sitting in a cave but my mind was in the city. I repeated all the prayers correctly, and people who heard them said they sounded wonderful. They admired how I would sit quietly for hours and hours in meditation. But nothing came to my heart. I didn't feel or realize anything.

When I saw the baby I understood my mistake, because I never cried, I never prayed sincerely, as the baby cried at the very end. I used to sit in prayer, but the moment I smelled some good food, I would finish quickly and go to the kitchen to eat. And when I sat down to pray, I would watch the time to make sure that I wouldn't be late for the first show. My prayers were not answered properly because they were not real and sincere.

Then I learned to pray for the sake of prayer and not for anything else. I would not be satisfied with anything but God. If our prayers are that sincere and our interest is only in God and nothing else, then God cannot sit quietly somewhere. He has to run to us. If we need help, it is always waiting. All we need to do is ask sincerely.

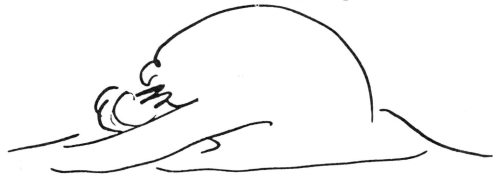

Help is not for the proud man. You must be like a baby; cry, ask for it. All of Nature is ready to give to you. You need not go and praise the sun to get light; just open the window and sunlight comes in. As long as you don't put up a barrier, you get light. Don't allow your pride to get between you and God's help.

Cry wholeheartedly, "Oh, Lord, help me. I can't do it by myself. I am so limited, so little." Let it be sincere. Let the eyes shed tears. Learn to cry well. Taste your tears. A hearty laugh or cry will relieve you from much tension. People who do not cry much have to go to the doctor very often. If you keep everything inside, it ferments.

When a child wants to show devotion to his mother, is there a restriction on how many times he should hug, how many kisses he should give? No. It comes automatically. Prayer, too, should be like that.

Of course, some people pray sincerely but ask for worldly things such as money or help on an exam. But even that is good because as their devotion develops, they think, "Why should I ask Him all these things? Won't He know what is good for me? He will give me everything that is necessary. He is all-knowing."

Then their prayers take a different turn. They say, "God, I don't need to ask. I might even ask for something that is not good for me. You know what is good. Just do what is proper. I don't know anything. All I need is faith and devotion to You." That is a much higher prayer.

Devotion gradually progresses to higher levels. The *Bhagavad Gita* talks about four kinds of devotees. One type goes to God and asks Him to remove his suffering. Another one will ask for money or material things. A third will request liberation or release from his bondage. And the fourth will not ask for anything. He will just enjoy praying and praising his Lord. That is the highest form of prayer.

People who don't believe in a God ask me, "Who is this God? Where is He? Is He hiding in a corner and pulling all the strings? What is the idea of prayer? Is God going to hear me and come running?"

To such people, I say that God is really everywhere, not in a particular form, but as an omnipresent awareness or power. God is consciousness itself. And by your concentrated, sincere prayer, you are tuning your mental radio to receive that power. If I say there is nice music in this room, some of you may disagree and say, "We don't hear any music. How can you say that there is music in the room?" To you, I say get a radio, tune it properly, and you will hear the music.

By tuning the radio, you are not creating music. It is already there; your tuning merely attracts the radio waves. If your tuning is not correct, if it moves a little off that particular wavelength, you won't receive the music. But the moment you find the correct wavelength, the music comes easily.

In the same way, you will receive God consciousness, God's grace, or the Cosmic Consciousness only when you tune your mind to the proper wavelength. Some people call that tuning "meditation," some call it "prayer," others call it "communion." Some say you need not do anything but sit quietly to go into that higher state. But even sitting quietly is doing something.

That God or Self or blissful pure consciousness is always there. You are not creating it by your meditation. You need not do anything to get into it, but you have to do something not to disturb that flow. We are not creating God's grace, but we are removing everything that prevents the grace from coming to us.

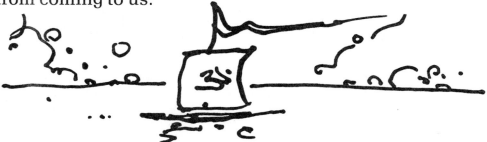

St. John begins his gospel, "In the beginning was the Word and the Word was with God and the Word was God." "The Word" can be understood to mean sound. In the beginning there was a sound, and that primal sound can be called God. Out of that sound, the whole universe was created.

Scientists say that the entire universe, what you see and what you cannot see, is nothing but atomic vibrations. When a dynamo starts rotating, the first thing you hear is a hum. The same with anything set in motion. When God, the static, unmanifested God, wanted to set Himself in motion, He hummed. In Sanskrit, the word for "individual self" is *hum.* In other words, we are all part of that cosmic hum.

Om, or the hum, is the basis of all the different sounds. Even if you honk a horn, it's nothing but the expression of Om. Stand on the beach, close your eyes, and listen to the music of the sea—it is Om. When the wind blows, it blows Om. When the fire burns well, you will get the same sound.

The elements themselves produce that sound. The movement of the elements is caused by Om. In other words, when the Om moves, it gives rise to the elements. The elements are not different from Om. Ultimately, everything is the expression of Om. It is the original sound.

When you realize the Truth, you are at home. Home is the place where you can be comfortable. Why is it called home? Because *om* is surrounded by *He. H* is on one side, *e* is on the other and *om* is right in the middle—you have God and His cosmic sound, so you feel at home.

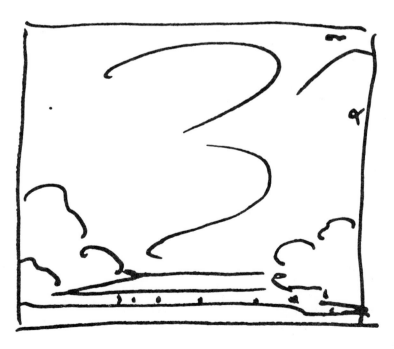

THE GURU
AND THE DISCIPLE

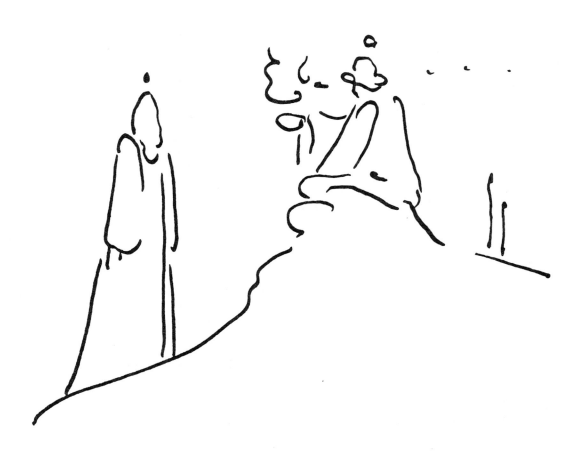

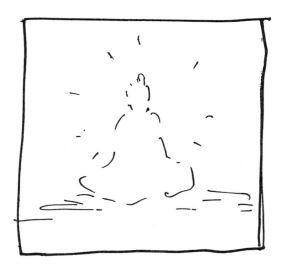

The term *guru* is very much used in America now, though sometimes sarcastically. Guru means the spiritual teacher. The guru is one who eliminates or removes the darkness in your understanding. The first syllable, *gu,* means darkness or ignorance, *ru* means the remover. So, one who removes the darkness is a guru.

His purpose is not simply to say, "You are wonderful." You may be wonderful but he will still say, "There is one black spot there. Correct it." A guru is nothing but a laundryman. He is trying to wash the dirty laundry.

Suppose you have a beautiful white shirt that has turned gray from all the dirt and dust it has accumulated. You give it to the laundryman to make it white again. But he doesn't really make it white. It is already a white shirt. All he does is remove the dirt so that we can see the whiteness again.

124

He scrubs it, soaks it, rinses it, wrings it, hangs it up to dry, and then irons it with a hot iron. When he gives it back to you, it is once again clean and beautiful. That is what the guru does with the mind of his student or disciple. He helps to clean it so its original purity can be seen.

Like the cloth, the mind undergoes a lot of suffering because of its stains. The more the stain, the more the pain. If it had never gotten stained, there wouldn't be any pain. Your mind was given to you fresh and pure, well made to suit your purpose, but somehow, you didn't take good care of it. You allowed it to run around and, by your wrong thoughts and actions, it accumulated all kinds of impurities.

When the mind is clean and uncolored from the accumulation of all this dirt, the True Self emerges. Liberation means being freed from the bondage of our own mind or ego. The ego doesn't want to accept anything. It will put a barrier between you and the teacher, so the teacher's first and foremost task is to see that the ego is cleaned. It is not destroyed but just made healthy. If the ego were destroyed, you would lose your individuality and incentive to learn.

To clean your mind, the teacher may ask you to do menial work. Actually, nothing is menial, but if he thinks it will deflate your ego, he will ask you to do it. His business is to take care of the ego. Once he sees that you are ready to do everything, then, even without your knowing, you start receiving.

There are a lot of "resistors" in us. We have to take out all the resistors, put in proper condensers, connect all the wires properly, and then the receiving set works well. If you know a little bit of electronics, you know that resistors are nothing but carbon sticks. Carbon is a burnt-out black substance. If the stick is a little too long, it won't allow anything to pass through.

In the same way, our system has many resistors. We have to undo them to clear the way. And ego creates the most resistance in you. Renouncing ego is very difficult. I will help by initiating you with the "ego mantram." It's easy. Every time you feel egoistic, say, "E-*go, e-go*." That's the ego mantram. It's nice, because the ego wants its name repeated. All right, say, "E-go! Get out!"

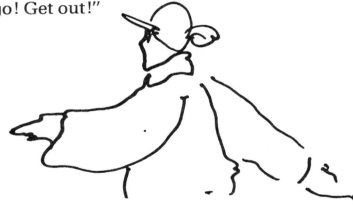

If you are capable, use your intelligence to analyze the qualifications of a realized person, a man of wisdom, an enlightened man, before you accept him as your guru. The signs of a man of wisdom are a settled mind, a steady mind, and a clear mind.

He will not run after anything. He will not be afraid of anything. He has no friend, no foe. Neither pleasure nor pain, profit nor loss, praise nor censure affect him. He is content, totally free from egoism and pride.

126

If you see such qualities in anybody, know that he is a sage. He is fit to be your guru. He is totally free from selfishness and ready to serve you at all times. At the same time, he won't force his service on you. Being a man of wisdom, he won't claim to be a realized man or the only realized man. Instead, he will be very humble. He will wait until you recognize him. If opportunity comes, he serves. If not, he waits.

A true teacher doesn't need advertisements. Have you ever seen a flower sending out a circular to all the bees saying, "I have honey, come to me?" No. When the flower is in bloom, all it has to do is be and the bees will come. When the tree is laden with fruits, it doesn't need to send invitations to the birds.

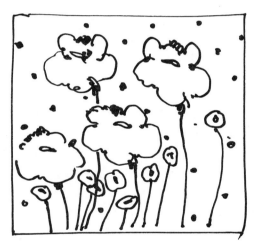

A guru will never call himself a guru. It is others who call him a guru. Ask Christ whether he created Christianity and he would say, "No. I don't know Christianity at all." Ask Buddha whether he created Buddhism and he would say, "I don't know Buddhism. All I know is the Truth." Followers create a cult. Great men never bottle their truth or label it for sale.

If you are attracted to a spiritual teacher, go, mingle with him and his followers, and see if you are satisfied. If you feel that you are getting help, follow him. But if he doesn't suit your taste, stay away. In a way, every teacher and every institution are necessary. They are all doing some service according to the will of the Lord.

We need all kinds of restaurants. If you like the food at one, go and eat there. If you don't like it, don't eat there, but don't criticize it. Someone else may like it. Just because you are allergic to tomato sauce, you don't need to condemn Italian food.

We should have an ecumenical approach. There is only one purpose in life—realizing the Self, peace, happiness, or God within. Whatever way you choose, as long as you get this, it's fine. There's a spiritual hunger and all the different teachers and institutions are spiritual restaurants.

If you follow the teaching of one individual, that doesn't mean all should follow him. The one and the same Spirit expresses itself in many forms and names to suit the age, time, and place. In one place the Spirit is called Jesus, in another place, Buddha. There's no need to claim that only one should be worshiped. They are all that one Spirit appearing as different men.

Small waves, big waves, foam, bubbles, spray, and icebergs are one and the same stuff in different forms. A little child welcomes a small wave. A daring fellow who wants to surf ignores the small waves and waits for big ones. Whichever you choose, see the sea behind them all. Then you become a seer.

If we understand the true Jesus to be the infinite essence, then we see that the same essence might have appeared in another name with a different body called Buddha. But the Spirit behind them is the same. When the ocean comes to one shore, it is called "Pacific." If it comes to another shore, it is called "Atlantic" or "Indian." Should we fight and say that the Pacific and Atlantic and Indian oceans have different waters?

No. The waters are the same, as is the Truth. It can appear in any form, under any name, at any time, to anybody. Whoever has eyes will see. Whoever has ears will hear.

The Ultimate Truth can be revealed only by somebody who has experienced it, who had it revealed to him by another person who had experienced it. No candle can light itself. Another lighted candle must come and touch it. That's the way Truth passes from person to person.

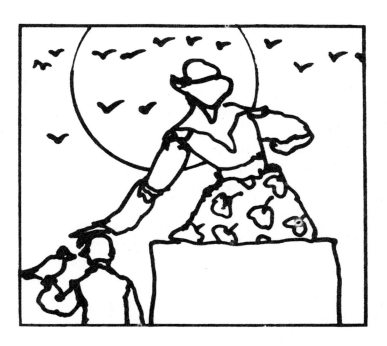

Often the role of the guru is misunderstood and the students think that the teacher will carry them to the goal. If you see a signpost that says BOSTON—200 MILES, do you prostrate yourself before the signpost, deck it with garlands, and pray, "Please take me to Boston?" No. The signpost simply points the direction and indicates the distance. You must do the walking.

The guru is like that. He has gone the route. He knows the journey and is able to guide others on the trip. But you have to follow the teaching. Even God cannot help you if you will not help yourself. The mind, looking for an easy way out, asks, "If God is all graceful and merciful, why doesn't He come and give me some grace and blessings?" The answer is that unless you seek, you will not find.

Many teachers or gurus are proclaimed by their devotees as a prophet or *Avatar.* If you recognize a guru as an Avatar, you will certainly be benefited by him. But there need not by only one Avatar. In fact, you are all Avatars. Avatar means God incarnate. You are all God incarnate. There is nothing less than God anywhere.

Everything is God. He didn't make the world out of something but out of Himself. That's why we say that He is omnipresent.

Wherever things are well polished, clean, and refined, you see a reflection. Essentially, we are all God, but somehow, not many of us seem to be reflecting or allowing that presence to be seen and felt. Those who feel themselves to be God incarnate and can also make others feel that way are called Avatars.

But they can't make everybody feel that way, because even to recognize an Avatar, one has to see with a certain clarity. Who will recognize a diamond? Only one with a knowledge of diamonds.

No guru will ever ask you to always be in his physical presence. That would create a dependence. Spiritual growth means freedom from bondage.

The teacher should liberate you. But in the beginning he may say, "Attach yourself to me so you can detach yourself from other things. And then I'll help you detach yourself from me also." If you want to go learn something somewhere else, he should say, "Fine, go." He won't feel that he is losing a disciple. He is more interested in your growth. If you feel you can learn more elsewhere, he will take you there himself.

A guru won't distinguish between people. He just gives. He sows seeds everywhere. Some will fall on rock, some on mud. Someday, a wind may blow the seed off the rock. He doesn't worry about that. His duty is to sow.

A holy man or guru never keeps anything for himself, everything passes through him. A flute has nothing inside and is full of holes. The flute allows the musician to play anything he wants through it. That's why it keeps itself completely empty and "holey."

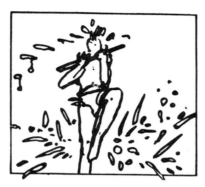

A guru never demands anything from you for teaching. While teaching, he learns. That is the lesson for the teacher. When Christ preached, he did not charge anything. His disciples would bring him food and he would distribute it to others. True spiritual teachings are always freely imparted.

But if you have something to give in return, offer it. There's no fixed fee. If you have a fruit, cut it into small pieces and offer a piece to the teacher. The student should go with some offering, but the teacher should not wait for it.

A guru will not force anything into you. He will wait until you ask, until you become ready. When you put total faith in him, that is the connection, the link. Once that trust is established, even if the guru refuses to teach you, you will learn from him because imparting true knowledge is not normally done with words. A guru may lecture for hours and hours, but it will be nothing compared with a minute of silent imparting.

By speaking through silence, in feelings, you can receive more than through words. True feeling will be limited by words. If someone says, "I love you, I love you," a hundred times a day, that is not loving you. He himself is doubtful of his love; that's why he tells you of it again and again. If love is there, why should he tell you? There is no need; you can feel it, it is something beyond words. His every look and action will be filled with it. It is a matter of feeling, not hearing. When the heart is full, the mouth closes automatically.

The Guru is eternal. The Guru never dies. It's only the physical body that dies. And what is a guru then? His words and teachings. They never die. Those truths are eternal. They are just transmitted to you through a physical body.

Ultimately, the guru makes you see the True Self or Guru within you. There are many disciples who rarely even see the Guru physically but still understand his lessons and teachings. That is possible when you really look within, meditate, and see him inside. Then you can get all the answers from within.

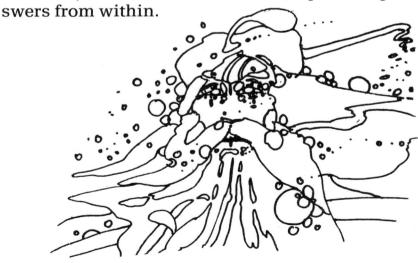

THE TRUE EDUCATION

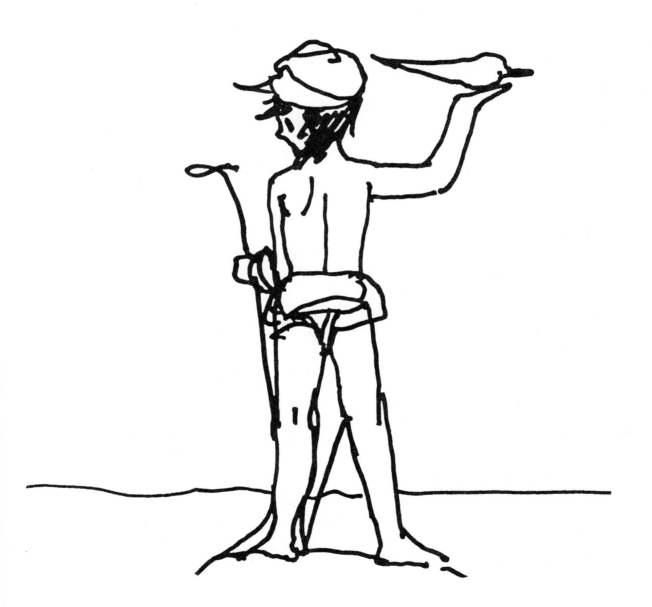

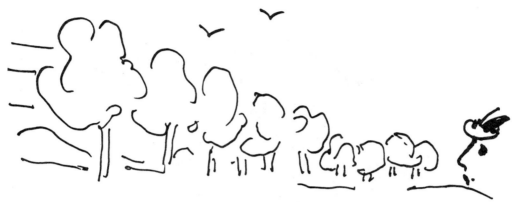

You have inborn qualities and the duty of the teacher is to bring them out. If an apple seed is sown, Mother Nature brings forth an apple tree, not an orange tree. In our modern schools, we bring in many different seeds and expect them all to be one kind of tree.

School should be a place where children develop their own identities and good qualities. The teacher should be ready to answer all questions. The teacher's duty is to answer questions, not to teach anything. When a child asks, "What is this?" the teacher should start the lesson. She can inject history, geography, chemistry, physics, philosophy, everything into her answer.

If a child picks up a banana and asks, "Where does it come from?" the teacher can talk about the banana plant, how it grows in what soil. Let the children pick up what they like. If they are tired and say, "I'm hungry," that becomes the eating lesson. Even while eating, the children can learn how to eat, how to use all their teeth, and how to chew.

136

The teacher can say, "Before you eat, think about how many people don't even have this much food today. Thank God for giving you this. If you have one banana and another person has nothing, share with him." There are many things that can be taught, even in eating. Let all of nature be the textbook.

Unfortunately, we don't see this very much in modern education. The teacher comes with his notes, stands in front of the class, and gives his lecture. It doesn't matter whether the students listen or not. The teacher finishes his job and goes away.

That's why education is becoming business. Teachers don't teach for the joy of teaching. They don't want to share their knowledge, they want to sell it. Most Indian village doctors feel that their medicine will not work if they sell it. It loses its spiritual quality and becomes a business. The doctor will never demand money. You have to find a way to pay him back. Sometimes that becomes a difficult job. You received something beautiful. He saved your life and you look for an opportunity to repay him. When he has to paint his house, many people will help him.

There is a bond of love between people that we call spirituality. Like the village doctor, a teacher should never expect anything in return for his knowledge. Knowledge is something like a well, where the more you draw from it, the more you get. If you are a doctor of medicine and don't practice for ten years, you will forget all you knew. Students help you maintain the knowledge that you gained so you must be thankful to them.

Gurus are all over. There is no scarcity of gurus. Anything and everything, anybody and everybody could be your guru. The really scarce commodity is the disciple. The scriptures say when the disciple is ready, the guru appears.

Once you accept a person as your guru, don't test him or see whether he says what you think he should say. To be a good disciple, you should first tell him, "I don't know anything. I trust you completely. Just tell me what to do." It's only then that the real guru-disciple relationship begins. Until then, it's just a friendly exchange.

Once a person went to a master and asked him for wisdom. He then tried to impress the master with all the wisdom that he already had. The master said, "Okay, I'll give you wisdom, but first have some tea." He began to pour the tea into the student's cup. He poured and poured until the cup overflowed and still he kept pouring.

Finally the student said, "Sir, my cup is full and you're still pouring. It's dripping onto the floor." "I know," said the master. "You, too, are already full. You have your own ideas and egoism. If I pour anything more—even the truth—there is no room for it in your cup. Go, empty the cup, and then come back."

If you take a pot half-filled with water, put it on your head, and walk, it will splash and make all kinds of noise. A full pot will make no sound at all. Any pot that makes too much noise is half-empty, remember that. If a person is full of knowledge, he will always say, "I don't know that much. I'm ready to learn a little more."

Everyone has something to give us. We don't lose anything by respecting others and being humble. To understand something, you have to stand under it. Humility, bowing down, is always good. Anything that has weight will bow down or bend over.

Look at a field of wheat. The minute it becomes ripe and heavy, it bends over. Nothing is lost by being humble and giving respect to others. Give respect and you get respect. Respect is like an echo. If you say, "Hello, my dear brother," you will get, "Hello, my dear brother," in return. If you say, "Hey, you stupid fool," you will get that back instead.

You get what you give. If you want respect, give respect. If you ever want to be a master, first become a good servant. Only a good servant will make a good master. You can never be a master without first being a servant. This is living philosophy. This is Yoga.

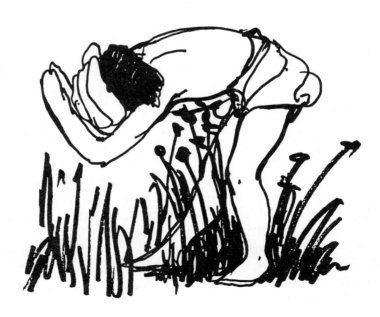

Many people do not want advice. If you say, "Put your finger in the flame and you will get burned," they say, "Why should I listen to you? It's none of your business." They want to experience things for themselves, so let them. The world will teach them the lessons they need.

Just be there, and if anybody comes and asks you something, tell them what you know. If people don't come and ask, don't go and tell them anything. Sometimes you may feel very sympathetic and feel like saying something. But wait. Look well and know for certain that they are ready to hear you, ready to listen.

Even then, don't demand that they accept your advice. Simply present it. "This is my feeling. This is my opinion. These are my reasons for believing it. If you like, try it. Otherwise, drop it."

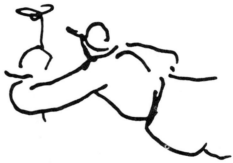

Have you ever seen a sparrow's nest? In India, they are big, bulblike things with two or three compartments, one below the other, hanging from one thread. Above is the living room and there's a bedroom down below. It's spun with thin fibers spliced from the palm leaf and all done by the beak. The whole thing faces downward, so when it rains, not even a drop can get in.

One rainy day, a sparrow was sitting in its comfortable

nest. When the rain stopped, the sparrow flew out and sat on the roof. He saw a monkey sitting on a branch nearby. When rain comes, a monkey doesn't have any nest so he just sits there getting drenched. You should see his sad face!

The sparrow looked at the poor monkey and said, "My brother, I feel so sorry for you. I have only a beak but look at this nice nest I made. You have four limbs and one tail, more than even a human being. You could have spent a little time building a house for yourself. Then you wouldn't be wet like this."

The monkey took it as teasing. "You have a nice home, that's why you didn't get wet, and now you come out and have the temerity to tease me. Well, watch what I'm going to do." With that, he jumped up and tore the nest to pieces. "Next rain, let us both get wet!"

There are people like that. If you say to them, "Hey, why don't you . . ." they get annoyed. So the best thing is to ignore them. They're not ready. Wait until they come and ask you. Until then, simply smile at them.

Even if they tease you and say, "What kind of people are you Yogis?" just say, "Well, we probably have a little screw loose somewhere, what can we do? You are clever and not involved in all this. What you are doing is fine."

Give them credit. A really intelligent man will simply call himself a fool if it is necessary. You don't need to prove that you are clever, that what you are doing is right. If you try to tell the wrong person the greatness of what you are doing, you are really proving that you are a fool. You should smile and say, "Well, we are just a little spaced out." Admit it.

You don't need to go and correct everybody. It's not your duty. Just take care of your peace. We're not here to reform the world.

Whenever you see happy people, show friendliness. When you see unhappy people, show compassion. When you see virtuous people, show joy. And when you see vicious people, ignore them. Don't try to teach them. They are not ready to take your advice. If you feel like saying something, say it gently, keeping an eye on how they are receiving what you say. If they are not receiving it well, stop and leave.

Silence saves you from quarrels. Many of our problems and enemies are created by our talking. Think of the times you were disturbed, the times you yelled at somebody and made enemies. You may well say, "I talked too much. If only I had learned to keep my lips shut, I could have avoided it." And if we stop talking, we save a lot of energy. People who talk a lot hear less. Nature has given you only one mouth but two ears.

Even so, we ignore the ears. We want others to use their ears while we use our mouth. The ears are always open. There is no door to the ear, but the mouth has well-built walls. Before any sound comes out, it has to pass through two rows of teeth and then through the lips. It's almost like a fortress.

Nature itself does this. So beware. Don't talk too much but be ever ready to listen.

A person must first know that he is in trouble before you can help him. Sometimes I get frantic calls from people saying, "Help me! I am doomed! I don't know what to do." That means they have realized their danger and want to change. It's easy to help them.

There is a saying. "One who knows that he knows not, help him. He's a good student, he's ready to learn. But one who knows not that he knows not, shun him, he's a fool. He's still not ready. One who knows that he knows, learn from him. He is a wise man."

If you mix milk and water and allow a swan to drink, it will drink only the milk. Swans can separate milk from water. The beak of the swan contains a chemical that curdles milk. The swan can easily drink the curdled milk, leaving the water behind. A good student is like the swan. He takes the useful things and leaves the unnecessary things behind.

Another type of student is like a parrot. You tell him something and he repeats it without digesting anything. Another student is a pot with many holes. You pour and pour but nothing remains inside. You talk to him for two hours and he looks at you, devouring every word. When he goes out and someone asks him, "What did Swami say?"

he retains nothing. Then there is another one, you can call him the tea strainer. When you pour tea on a strainer, the nice tea passes through and the strainer retains only the dirt.

The *Bhagavad Gita* describes a good disciple by saying: "He who hates no being, who is friendly and compassionate to all, who is free from the feeling of I and mine, even-minded in pain and pleasure, and forebearing; ever content, steady in meditation, self-controlled, and possessed of firm conviction, with mind and intellect fixed on Me, he, My devotee, is dear to Me."

"By whom the world is not affected, and whom the world cannot afflict, he who is free from joy, anger, fear and anxiety, he is dear to Me."

"He who neither rejoices, nor hates, nor grieves, nor desires, renouncing good and evil, full of devotion, he is dear to Me."

"He who is the same to friend and foe, and also in honor and dishonor, who is the same in cold and heat, in pleasure and pain, who is free from attachment, to whom censure and praise are equal, who is silent, content with anything, homeless, steady-minded, full of devotion—that man is dear to Me."

Disciplehood is very difficult to achieve because it needs wholehearted faith, devotion, and intelligent discrimination. Let us all be good disciples. Let no one think that he has learned all, because there is no end to learning. As long as we learn, we are disciples. Let us always learn and grow.

Who will find supreme peace? One who practices with complete faith, one who has that total interest and zeal. When even an atom of doubt gets into you, your first and foremost duty is to remove it. Doubt is like a drop of poison falling into a pot of nectar, spoiling the whole pot. Doubt in anything poisons it, be it friendship, family, business, or your relationship with the guru.

If you know the cause of your doubt, go and ask the person about whom you have the doubt. Talk about it. Don't keep it in your mind. It's always better to question and resolve it. If you suspect somebody, every action will add to your suspicion. That's why doubt should be cleared up as soon as possible.

Recently, somebody told me, "I love you and want to follow you and your teachings but still have my doubts." It's contradictory. If you love something, you can't have doubt. If you have doubt about the very thing that you are doing, how can you love it? Can you say, "I love you but I still have a little doubt about you?" It's not love then. If you cannot clear up your doubt, find somebody else. Otherwise, you are wasting your time.

Doubt of your own actions means that you lack confidence in what you are doing. If you don't know whether what you are doing is right or wrong, you should probably consult someone who does know. The doubt must be cleared up at all costs. There's nothing wrong with having doubts, but don't allow them to continue.

Suppose you are walking on a road and you see a fork. You don't know which way to go so you just sit there and wonder. Then you are going nowhere. You should have the courage to ask someone if he knows the way and then try one of the paths. You may not be sure, but at least it's worth a try. If you reach a dead end, you can come back and go the other way.

Either believe in your own judgment and do something, or believe in others' judgment. If you do not have either of these beliefs, you stagnate. You can't go anywhere.

Be convinced before you do something. Don't do anything just for the guru's sake, however beautiful it is.

If someone can convince me that smoking grass will give me a golden key to heaven, I am ready to smoke it today. But convince me first. I am not just blindly saying no. If you can convince me that by eating some meat I will enjoy perfect health, I'll do it.

Buddha clearly said, "Please don't accept something because I said it or because the books say so." Are you convinced of it? If you are convinced, it becomes yours, then it is easy for you to follow. One's own experience is the best teacher.

Always wait and listen. Learn from experience. Your school education alone will not bring all your knowledge. Learn in the universal university. Learn from your daily life.

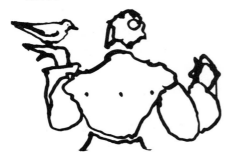

When you know where you stand, it's easy for you to know other things and their positions. If you know that you are in New York, then you can call California "the west." If you're in Japan, California becomes east.

This is subjective or relative knowledge. Know where you are, then you will know your relationship to other things. But there is also absolute knowledge, where there is no relativity because there is only One. Knowing that One, you know the essence of everything, the Fundamental Truth.

I don't say that if you know that One, you will know how to drive a car. That's a relative thing to be learned separately. But you will know the essence of which the car is made.

The Fundamental Truth is not something that somebody can give you. If somebody gives it to you one day, somebody can rob you of it the next. Even with God, it's not that you reach God or get God, but you *realize* God. You know that He is already there.

When I was a young student, I won a prize in an elocution contest—a bundle of big, heavy books. I opened them and they were all philosophy, no good stories or pictures, just Greek and Latin. I was discouraged and disappointed but I kept them, just to show that I had won.

Seven years later, I had a fever and had to lie in bed. The doctor asked me not to go anywhere and there was no work to do. Somehow my interest turned toward the books. I opened them and they were a great wealth for me then. I was able to understand every line, and I praised the people who had selected them for me.

What you do not appreciate today might be very useful tomorrow. I used to tell children, "Keep a thing for ten years and you will find a use for it." Paper clips, pens, I always find a use for them after some months. If that is so with even tiny things, how can we ignore and throw away age-old traditions and practices?

Sometimes we have to modify certain practices according to the age without leaving the Truth behind. But if the principle is forgotten, any ritual or practice is meaningless. Rituals are the outcome of certain basic principles. Do not shun something because you do not understand it or because old people are doing it. Keep it aside and one day you may be able to make use of it.

A young plant needs a fence around it. It cannot say, "Why do you put me in prison? I don't want to be inside here." Suppose the farmer says, "If you want, I'll remove the fence." The next minute, the cattle will come and chew the plant up.

Accept disciplines until you grow into a tree. Once the tree has grown up, there is no need for a fence, and that same tree will give shelter and shade to the cattle who would have eaten it earlier. As a young plant, you need discipline for your own protection; as a grown tree, you are free to protect others.

When a fruit is still green, it clings to the branch of the tree. If you try to pull it off, it refuses to come. That means it's not ripe yet. It still wants to be with the tree. So, imagine you are a fruit like that. As long as you are green, you want to stick to the tree of life. You can't jump off; you can't even allow somebody to pull you off. If by any chance you are pulled, you get hurt. If somebody pulls you off prematurely, even at your request, you are not fit to eat.

Instead, stick to the tree. Gather all the nourishment that you can get from the tree, because the tree of life is there to give you experience. When you get everything and are fully ripe, even before you think of it, you just drop off. The tree pushes you off instead of you pushing the tree. That means you are a dropout from the tree of life. Such a person will never fear the experiences of life.

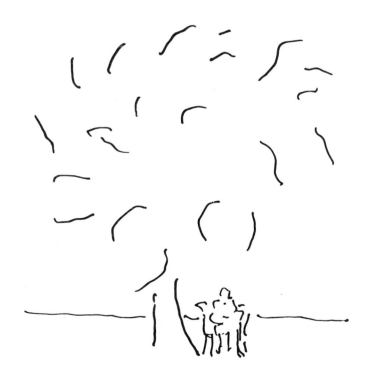

SELFLESSNESS

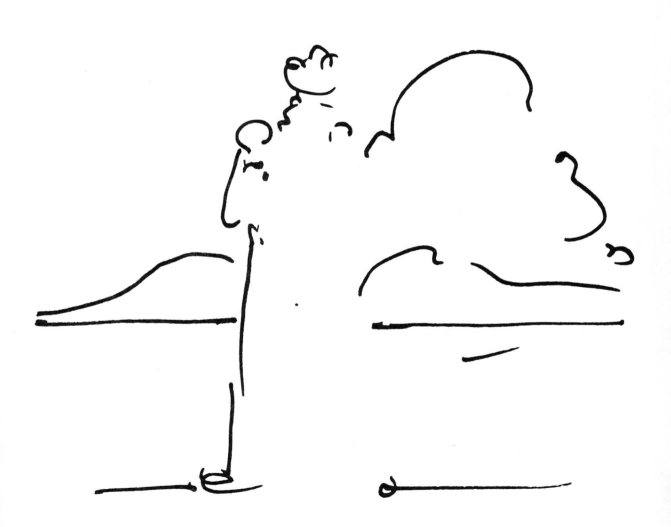

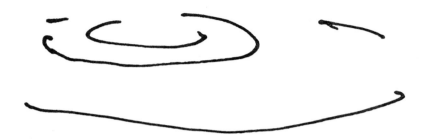

If you dam up a river, it stagnates. Running water is beautiful water. So be a channel. If anything comes, pass it on. Don't cling.

If you are not selfish, you can never be restless. Nobody can upset you, nobody can disturb you, I guarantee it. No selfish man can ever find peace and no selfless man can ever be irritated, upset, or disturbed.

Anytime you feel even a little bit disturbed, sit quietly and ask, "Why am I disturbed? What is the reason?" Don't try to blame somebody else. Ask yourself if you had an expectation for something to happen. When you want something to happen and it doesn't, you get upset. "I loved him so much but he didn't love me back so I'm upset." Here you lost two things: you lost his love and your peace of mind.

The selfish man always loses twice. If you think instead, "I am loving for the sake of love because loving makes me happy," that happiness cannot be taken away by anybody. It isn't based on somebody doing something or something that may happen later. That is contentment.

Enjoy the happiness of giving. Don't disturb it by expecting anything, even thanks. If you don't receive thanks, you lose the happiness of having given. And who is the cause for your disturbance? You.

What is the cause for disappointment? Your appointments. Simple enough. When an appointment is disturbed, it's called a "dis-appointment."

When you act, if you have a personal motive or if you expect a reward, you build up a tension even before you start. There is expectation, and anxiety. There is fear of losing something. Instead, if the mind is kept free from any expectation whatsoever, and your action is done just for the sake of action, for the sake of others, then that action is a perfect one.

If the results of an action bring benefit to all people concerned, without bringing harm to anybody, then it is a perfect action. But if it brings harm even to one individual, or if it builds up a tension in your own mind, it's not a perfect action. If you give ten dollars to somebody who is standing near a bar, you can't call it help. If a mother feeds her child all the candy it wants to eat, she's not helping the child. In each of these cases, giving is causing harm to someone.

If you are not sure if you should do something, ask yourself whether you are doing it for selfish reasons or for the benefit of others. If it's for selfish reasons, you may often go wrong. But if it is for the benefit of others, you will never go wrong.

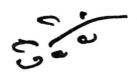

Sometimes even telling a lie may be a selfless and perfect act. It is the outcome that is important. Once upon a time there was a *sadhu,* a hermit, who lived in a remote, rural place. He led a very quiet life, praying and meditating. One evening, he was sitting outside his hut when all of a sudden he saw a beautiful young girl wearing costly jewels, running toward him crying, "Please save me! There's somebody chasing me who wants to kill me and steal my jewels!"

Then, without even waiting for his permission, she hid herself inside his hut. Within a few minutes, a wild-looking man with a dagger in his hand ran up saying, "Did you see a girl come this way?" What should the hermit have done? Should he have been honest and said, "I always tell the truth. The girl is hiding inside."?

No. Instead, he said, "What girl? Do you think a young, beautiful girl would come to this hermitage? Nobody like that ever comes here."
"Okay," said the man with the dagger, "I'm going to look for her in the other direction." Then he ran on.

By telling a lie, three lives were saved. The man would have killed the girl and, not wanting to leave the hermit as a witness, he would have killed him as well. When he went to pawn the jewels, the police would have caught him and he would probably have been hanged. Three lives would have been lost because of the hermits honesty so the motive and the outcome should be thought of in every action, not just the action itself.

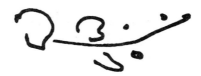

A papa was carrying his child in one arm and a package in the other when the child said, "Papa let me hold your package so that you will be carrying less." The papa laughed and gave the package to the child.

Ultimately, everything is being carried by God but childish or egoistic people still like to carry things themselves. The ego says, "I have to do it for myself." Fine, do it, and when you do it, you will become responsible for it.

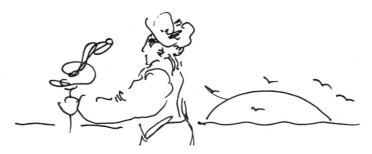

That is what we call *karma.* You do something by yourself, for your sake and you have to face the result. If you do something instead for God's sake, for the benefit of humanity in His name, without the least personal expectation, it becomes Karma Yoga. The benefit might come, but we don't expect it. There is no personal motivation. In Karma Yoga, you are free from the results, either pleasure or pain, virtue or demerit.

The minute you want something for your sake, you are restless until you get it. Once you get it, you are still not really happy because you don't want to lose it. If you do not get it, you feel anger, hatred, and enmity.

You believe that somebody else is the cause of your not getting it; you blame somebody. You say, "That fellow got in my way, otherwise I would have gotten it." You create enemies around you.

But if your want is not for your sake, you don't worry about the result. It's not your profit or loss. Eliminate selfishness from your life. The minute you decide to lead a selfless life, eternal happiness is yours.

If you do something and think, "*I* want the prize. *I* have done it. *I* must be honored. *I* will do it. *I* will get it," all your actions, and their reactions, are colored by your thoughts and desires. The more desires, the more colors or dirt they accumulate.

The God in you is like an all-consuming flame, eternally burning. If you put dirt on it, the dirt will get burned. Unfortunately, you don't allow the dirt to fall on God but want to keep it for yourself. You have a chimney around the flame, your mind, and it accumulates all the dirt.

But when dirt comes, if you say, "I don't want it. Let me offer it to God," what happens? If you allow the dirt to fall right on the flame inside, it will burn. Don't keep it for yourself. If you keep it for yourself, you neither know how to burn it nor how to digest it. You get covered by it.

Do everything in the name of God and nothing will affect you. Say, "Let me not use the will I have been given to carry unnecessary burdens. Let me use my will to realize Your will." Then you become a beautiful instrument in the hands of the Lord. The light, the flame, reflects through your chimney. If the chimney is colored and crooked, you get colored and distorted light. So make the chimney clean and free from all color. Once the chimney is made crystal clear, you see the inner light shining.

Someone once asked me, "When I do things for others, that's Karma Yoga, but when I work and get a salary, can I think of that as Karma Yoga also?" Yes. What are you going to do with your salary? Why do you want to live in a house? Why do you want to eat? Why do you want to love? To serve others. Isn't it so?

How can you serve without eating? You have to fill up the tank so that the car will move. You have to keep it tuned up and washed. You have to have a garage for it. So, too, you have to have a garage and fuel for this body, and how can you do that without money? With money, you prepare and equip yourself with enough energy to give energy back.

Even your eating, sleeping, and drinking become Karma Yoga if you do them selflessly, thinking, "I am only keeping myself fit to serve others. If I am not going to serve others, I don't need to eat, I don't need to sleep, I don't need to have a house, I don't even need to live."

If you serve others and your salary is not enough to take care of your day-to-day expenses, you can even demand more. With that money, you are not just enjoying yourself. You are not simply satisfying your senses. You are not overindulging in anything. You are just taking good care of yourself and others who are under your care. That is also part of your duty.

If you are living for the sake of everybody, serving God and His creation every minute with every breath, you are worshiping constantly. Work becomes worship and every act is a part of that worship.

If you ask a plant,"What is your purpose? Why did you blossom? Why are you here?" it will tell you, "I don't know. I just blossomed. And now I am being used. I am decorating the table." That's the purpose of the flower. It grows, gives out a nice fragrance, is beautiful, and dies when its allotted time is over.

Likewise, everything on this earth has a purpose, and that purpose is to serve, to be useful, and to bring some benefit to somebody. Wherever you look, you see giving. There's no asking. Take an apple tree. Does it demand that you give it water? Does it demand that you fertilize it? No. It doesn't demand anything.

Ultimately, with much hardship, it brings forth fruit. It would be reasonable for the tree to claim all the fruit for itself, but have you ever seen an apple tree tasting its own fruit? It gives not only to the people who praise it but to those who stone it. If somebody threw a stone at you, would you give him ten dollars? No. You would sue him for a hundred dollars!

Sacrifice is the law of life. A candle burns and we make use of the light while it slowly dies. An incense stick gives us fragrance while becoming ash. Humans claim to be the highest species but we could learn a lesson from the tree, the candle, and the incense stick.

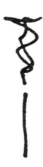

Sorrow is nothing but what you borrow. The cause of our suffering is our wrong approach—our greed, our attachment, and our clinging to things. The more we are attached to things, the more we suffer. Have you ever seen a silk moth? A silk moth is fed on mulberry leaves. A tiny moth becomes as big as your thumb within thirty or forty days by continuously eating. Day and night it eats and eats and eats. And, as you all know, when you eat a lot you get tired. You feel drowsy and you go to sleep. Normally when you go to sleep with a heavy, heavy stomach you dream. So the moth, after so much eating, goes to sleep and starts dreaming.

While rolling around and dreaming, the excess stuff that it ate passes out through its mouth as a thick, pasty string. The moth dreams and rolls continuously and the string becomes a cocoon. Then it enters a very deep sleep while the cocoon dries and becomes a strong fortress.

When the silk moth opens its eyes after its sleep, it sees itself caught in a cage. It wonders, "What happened to me? Why am I like this?" Then it recollects, "Yes, I started eating and I ate and ate and ate. I never gave anything to anybody. Everything I got I ate myself. Because of this, I fell into a dream of ignorance and now I am caught in it. Now I understand. It's my greed, my clinging onto things that brought me this cage. It's a self-made fetter, a self-made bondage."

Thus dispassion dawns in its life, and with it, wisdom. With the help of the wings of wisdom and dispassion and the small, sharp nose of intellect, it is able to escape from the cage, look back and laugh at it, then fly away, never to return.

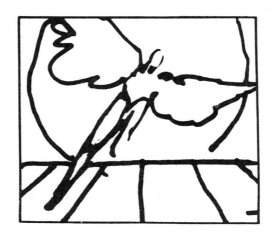

People also are like this. They never say no to things. They acquire more and more. Ultimately, they see that they are bound by their possessions. If they are fortunate, wisdom dawns and they get the dispassion to see that their suffering is self-made. Nobody on earth can make us suffer. Suffering is caused by our own attitude and our own ignorance. We think that by acquiring things we can be happy, and ultimately, these same things are what make us more unhappy.

There's nothing wrong in having things. Have them, but not for the sake of finding happiness. Have them to use for the sake of humanity. In an office, there are many things: a chair, a table, a typewriter, and a telephone. They are all for your use while you work there. When you walk out, you can't take them with you.

The entire world and the things in it are for our use, not for our possession. We have forgotten how to use the world and, instead, expect happiness to come from it.

Poverty is not giving up possessions and calling yourself poor, wearing rags, leaving your mansion, and living in a tepee saying, "I am growing spiritually." I have seen such tepees. When I went to visit one, the people living there said, "Isn't it a beautiful tepee! Please don't touch it!"

They renounced their palace but are clinging onto their tepee. It's like renouncing expensive suits and then becoming attached to patched-up old jeans. Renunciation means having the proper attitude. If you detach yourself mentally, you can keep the whole world around you. It will never affect you.

A bank teller handles millions of dollars. If he identified himself with the money, he would call himself a millionaire. He never identifies himself with it, but at the same time, has a duty toward it.

Fulfill the duty but don't be attached. Once you lose yourself in your attachments, you are affected by them and can't handle them properly. If an electrician puts on gloves before handling a live wire, he can use it and not be affected by it. Mental detachment is a kind of insulation. You insulate yourself with the attitude that "nothing belongs to me but I have a duty toward everything—my family, my country, my neighbor, and the world at large."

Everything, even your body, is given to you for your use, not just to possess. If a vehicle is given to you, take good care of it. Use the proper fuel. If it is made for high octane, don't use regular gas. When you use things, you have a responsibility to leave them clean and in good working order. Don't think that because they're not yours, you can do anything to them.

Detachment in action does not imply irresponsibility. When you do anything, you are totally responsible for it. You have even more responsibility in selfless action than in selfish action. In selfish action, if you are irresponsible, it is your loss. But in serving others, if you are irresponsible, many people lose.

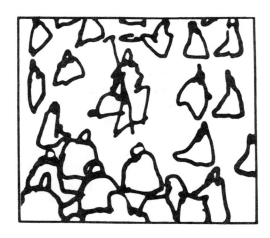

Detachment keeps your mind calm and serene. The moment you show any attachment, you put tension in the mind. An eminent surgeon can perform any kind of operation with ease, but for even a small operation on his wife, he gets nervous and calls in another doctor. A shaking hand can never perform an operation. An action is an operation and you can't operate on anything if you shake, mentally or physically. People are nervous because they are selfish. A selfless man need never be nervous.

Every morning many people check their weight by standing on a scale. Before they get on, they check whether the balance needle is at the zero point. If it fails to register at zero, their weight will be incorrect. In the same way, when we want to weigh things and pass judgment, we have to do it from a neutral point.

Take the case of a trial judge. If a person on trial is his relative, the case is transferred to another court because, unconsciously, there will be a prejudice and the judgment may not be correct. The neutral point can be achieved only by a completely detached mind. Yoga is neutrality, tranquility, and equanimity.

Once a King went into a forest where he saw a Swami sitting. The King said, "I have never seen such a joyful person. You are a great saint." He fell at his feet and said, "Come with me to my palace for a while." The Swami said, "What would I do in a palace? The whole world is my palace." "Please come," said the King, "just to make me happy." "Okay," said the Swami, "to make you happy, I'll come."

They arrived at the palace and went to a beautiful meditation room. The King wanted to show the Swami that he was a great devotee. He wanted to demonstrate his capacities so he sat at his altar and said proudly, "I normally do at least an hour of meditation. Will you excuse me?"

He then did his meditation and all kinds of pranayama, praying and chanting. You know how you do better when somebody's watching you. It's a "demon-stration." You demonstrate because the demon of pride is there. But toward the end of the King's meditation his real motives emerged. The King prayed, "God, the only thing I want is that little country next to mine. I'm going to wage a war against it, so please grant me a victory."

When he finished his meditation, he saw the Swami walking towards the door. "Swami, Swami," he called, "where are you going?" "Back to the forest," said the Swami, "I'm not used to staying with beggars." "Beggars!" said the King, insulted, "I am the King, I have everything." "No you don't," said the Swami, "you wanted a little more. As long as you still want something more and you beg of God, you are a beggar."

There once were three thieves who lived in a village on the banks of a river. At one time they were successful thieves, but then everyone in the village caught on to them. Whenever something was stolen, the people in the village knew where to look for it.

The thieves began to realize that crime doesn't pay. They repented for their past life and decided to start out fresh as honest people. But even though they wanted to leave their past behind, their reputation followed them.

The only thing left to do, they decided, was to go to another village where nobody knew them. There they would be able to make a fresh start. They packed their bags and went down to the banks of the river because most travel in those days was done by boat.

When they arrived at the river, they realized that they had no money with which to rent a boat. So they sat down to think of a plan. "I have it!" said one of the thieves after some time. "We will wait until it gets dark, and then steal one of the boats. What is one more crime when we have already committed so many? We will just postpone our honesty for one more day." They all agreed it was an excellent plan and waited for night.

That night they quietly boarded a boat and began to row. They took great care to row very quietly and rowed all night long. As the sun rose in the morning, they saw a village very similar to the one they had just left.

A man came running down to the shore raising his fist at them. "Hey, you thieves," he shouted, "where do you think you're going?" They were puzzled. How did he know they were thieves? How could their reputation have spread this fast?

"We are honest men," they replied. "We have just come from another village." "You are thieves!" he shouted back at them. "You have stolen my boat." This really had them confused. "How could this be your boat?" they inquired. "We have been rowing all night from another village."

The man laughed at them. "Not only are you thieves, but you are fools as well. How did you expect to get anywhere? You forgot to untie the boat from the dock!"

If you really want to get ahead in this river of life, you have to cut loose the ties that bind you. You can't reach your goal unless your bonds are removed. Unfortunately, our boats have thousands of anchors.

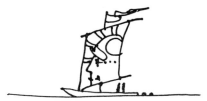

Everything that you call "mine" is holding you. If you want to know how far away you are from your goal—call it God or peace—write down everything that you call "mine": my house, my body, my intelligence, my child, my wife, my money, my country, my this, my that.

When there is nothing for you to call "mine," you are there. That's all. It's very simple. You don't need to practice anything.

If you really want peace, the simplest way is to make a checklist: How many "mines" have I put around me? The more mines around you, the more you are in trouble. Because every mine is ready to explode. You are making life a battlefield, burying mines everywhere.

If you have already buried them, call a good minesweeper or mind-sweeper. He will know how to defuse your mines. Once the fuses are gone, there won't be confusion. How will he remove the fuses? He will change the label from all that you call "mine" to "Thine."

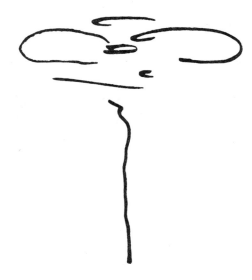

If you run after things, they will bring you anxiety, worry, and fear. The greater your position, the thicker the bullet-proof glass in your windshield. You create your own prison. The more you acquire and the harder you work to acquire it, the more you fear losing it.

Try running after your shadow. The faster you run, the faster your shadow runs ahead of you. And that's what happens when people try to get happiness from outside themselves. When they get tired of running, they say, "All right, I know I can't catch my shadow. I don't even want to." A kind of detachment dawns. They turn around to walk back and that same shadow they were running after is following them.

That's the secret in life. If you run after things, nothing will come to you. But if you are content and don't want anything, things will say, "Here is a man who never bothers us, who never chases us, so let's go and be with him." They know that you are not going to catch them and imprison them. They will be with you for as long as they want. When they want to go, they will leave and you won't be concerned.

If you run after power, position, fame, or money, you are not going to get them. If by some chance you do, you are not going to be happy. Let things run after you. The sea never sends an invitation to the rivers. That's why they run to the sea. The sea is content. It doesn't want anything.

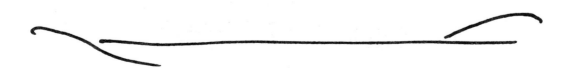

If anything good comes, know that it comes from God. Be grateful to Him or Her or whatever name you want to use. Become a good instrument in God's hands and leave the entire burden on His shoulders.

He will prompt you. He will tell you what to do and when to do it. Don't worry about tomorrow day after day. Live today well, with all ease. We have to plan for tomorrow, so plan for it. But know that your plan is just your plan and it will go through only if God says okay. Plan pending approval. If God approves, go do it. If it doesn't happen, know that He didn't approve and that's fine also.

At night when you lie down, you are lying down to sleep, not to plan for tomorrow. Forget the world and be like a baby. Think, "Mama, I am just putting my head in your lap. Take care of me. If you want me to get up tomorrow and do some work, wake me."

Every day we die. The following morning we are born again. Think that way and your sleep will be wonderful.

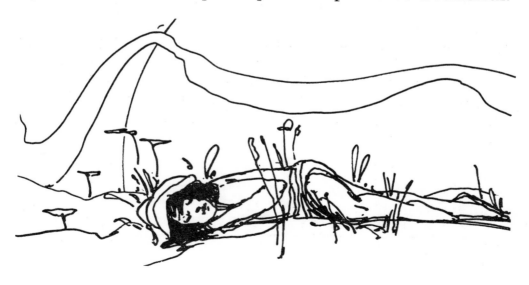

Finish the day's job and say, "I worked to my capacity. If there is anything wrong, it's due to my weakness. Anything good is due to the intelligence given to me. These are my accounts for the day. I am closing my shop."

Like a cashier in a bank, put everything in the safe and take the key. Think, "I am going home. If I am still alive tomorrow, I will come back to the job."

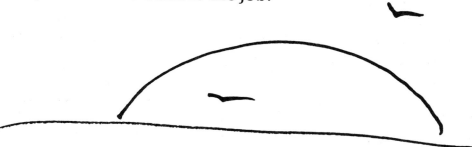

If you keep giving, the world will take care of you. If a cow gives milk, the farmer will take care of it. If it doesn't give milk, he will dispose of it. If a tree brings forth a lot of fruit, we water it, nourish it, and put a fence around it. But if it's not bearing any fruit, we chop it down.

So you don't need to worry about taking care of yourself. Just keep giving, and the world will want to receive more. It will take good care of you. But if people don't want to take care of you, if you are a burden to them and can't be useful, say good-bye and go. Let your place be occupied by somebody else.

A man who is totally free from wanting will be wanted by the Higher Will. He will be taken over by that Higher Will through friends and other people. Your car doesn't need to worry about filling itself with gas or oil. The worry is yours because you want to use it. The car never asks you to fill it up.

Don't think that by giving yourself completely you are losing yourself. When a drop gives itself completely to the sea, can you say the drop has lost itself? Maybe the drop lost its name *drop*. It dropped out as a drop. But it dropped in to become the sea.

Drop in. Don't be dropouts. Drop into that universality. Don't make yourself a separate drop or separate bits and pieces. The more that you think you are a bit, the more you will become bitter. The more you think you are a piece, the more peace you will lose.

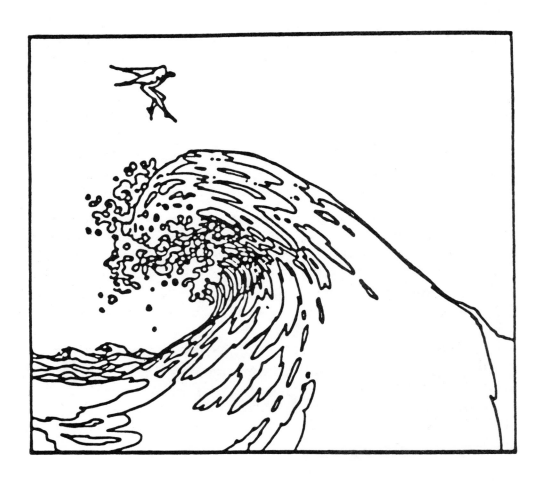

A man once went to an ashram seeking enlightenment. He bowed down before the Swami and said, "I'm interested in knowing the Self. I want to find peace. Please give me this wisdom." The Swami smiled at him and said, "Poor man, you are going to die in ten days. It's too late."

The man was shocked. "You mean that I'm really going to die in ten days?" "Yes. I see Death coming to you. He's very close." "What am I to do, Swami? Is there anything you can teach me?" "It's not that easy. Many people practice for years and still haven't found the wisdom."

The man kept on asking so the Swami finally said, "Okay, go home, and if by chance you live longer than ten days, come back to me. Then I will teach you. I could be wrong. If you don't die, come back."

The man returned home in a sad mood. Some friends came to see him and asked, "Why are you looking so sad?" "Well, the Swami at the ashram said that I will die within ten days. I really don't know what to do. I have committed many sins and I don't know how to atone for them."

At that moment, the man who kept his accounts came and said, "Sir, we have to sue that man who owes you money." But the man answered, "Forget about it. I loaned him money because I have enough. If I hadn't enough for my own expenses, I wouldn't have given him the loan. If he can't pay it back now, what's the use of sending him to jail? If he pays, all right. Otherwise, tell him that I erase the debt. He can enjoy the money." The accountant was very surprised because the previous day the man had told him to fight the case and to demand full payment and compound interest.

Then the man called his brother, to whom he had not spoken in ten years. The brother was surprised because the man had once told him that he would treat him as his deadly enemy. So he came with much hesitation. But the man who was going to die embraced him and said, "Brother, forgive me. I have misunderstood you all these years. Let's forget our enmity and become brothers and friends again."

Then, one after another, he started calling his enemies and making friends with them. The next day, he called the accountant, discovered he had a lot of money in the bank, and started writing checks. He knew that when he died, his children would waste the money on foolish things, so he left just a little in the bank for their education. With all the rest, he wrote checks to different institutions and worthy groups. They took the money and started helping the sick and feeding the poor.

The world wondered, "What's happening to him? All of a sudden he's really becoming a big, broad-minded man. He's making friends with everyone and giving everything to charity." But no one knew he was to die in a few days.

Now there were just two days left. The worry made him unable even to eat and he became very weak. He became sickly and had to stay in his bed. He'd learned some Yoga and didn't differentiate among religions so he asked a Catholic monk to read the Bible, a Hindu monk to read the *Gita,* and the Yogis to come and chant. His idea was to hear as many nice prayers as possible before he died.

By now, the whole town had come to know of him and everybody was praising him. His name was in all the headlines. The tenth day came and he told everyone, "I've finished my work. Don't bother me anymore. I'm going to sit down and meditate." He started repeating a mantram—and waited for Death to come.

He looked at his watch. It was midnight of the tenth day. He thought something had gone wrong. The Swami said ten days. He asked the servants to check the doors. They were unlocked so that Death could have easily entered.

Even though he felt weak, he called some friends and asked them, "Please take me to the Swami." By that time there were hundreds of people willing to do anything he asked. When they arrived at the ashram, he went to the Swami, fell down at his feet, and said, "Swami, what has happened? Your prediction went wrong. I didn't die." "Yes, I see that you didn't die. Something must have gone wrong somewhere. The Lord of Death was probably just delayed. Wait here for another day and see if he comes. If he doesn't come, I will teach you."

So, he sat in a room and meditated. The eleventh day also passed. He got up and said, "Swami, I'm still alive. Death hasn't come. At least now, please teach me the wisdom." The Swami smiled at him and said, "I've already taught you." "What?" said the man. "You didn't teach me anything. I don't understand."

"All right," said the Swami. "What have you been doing for the last ten days? How many lies did you tell? How many people did you murder? How many enemies did you make? How much black-market business did you do?"
"Swami, how could I do any of those things? I made up

with all my enemies and gave away everything to charity. I became a very good man because there was no time to waste. I knew I was going to die, and I didn't want to die with a bad name, so I patched up everything."

"What did others think of you before?" "Nobody liked me. They said I was good for nothing, that I was a very bad man." "And now, what do they say?" "When I leave the house, everybody praises me and there are many articles in the paper. They all seem to like me. They call me a great, saintly man."

"Are you happy about it?" "Yes, Swami. Absolutely. I'm happy when everybody likes me and I like everybody." "Fine, then, go back home, know that you may die any minute, and don't make anyone your enemy. Live the same way you have been doing these past ten days. That is the essence of Yoga. Then you will always know peace. That is wisdom."

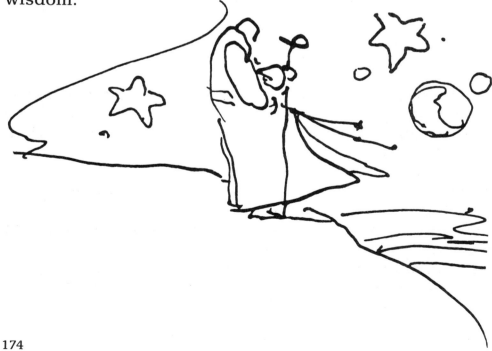

Do we know when we are going to die? No, it can happen any minute. So why create enemies? Why tell lies? Live the Golden Rule as best you can. Be nice to everybody. Serve all without any discrimination whatsoever.

"Let me be useful to everybody. Let my entire life be a sacrifice for humanity." This is the secret of Yoga. If you lead a life like this, peace and joy will come automatically. But without such a life, all your Yoga postures, breathing, chanting, and meditation will be of no use. They'll be rituals without any meaning, decorations for a lifeless body. What is the use of decorating a corpse? Only with the proper understanding is it worth having a healthy body and a sound mind.

Businessmen, do fair business. People who work in different industries and factories, work for the sake of everyone. Professional people, don't just sell your knowledge; serve one another well.

Instead of talking about peace and joy, about God, how great He is, or where He is, do something to realize Him. Keep the mind clean. The only requirement to see that peace or joy or God, whatever name you use, is a clean, peaceful mind. Stay away from anything that disturbs your peace of mind, from anything that brings disappointments, anxieties, and worries.

This means questioning, "I'm going to steal. Will that keep my mind clean? Am I selfish in doing it?" If the answer is yes to the first question and no to the second, you will keep your mind clean. You are not selfish. I really mean that. You can even steal without being selfish.

If somebody wants to commit suicide, hides a little cyanide under his pillow, and you steal it, is that selfish? I have done it, so I am a thief, but I am happy I did it. It's not what you do that is important, but why you do it and what the outcome is.

Put others first. Only then will you really find peace and joy. The people we call great saints and prophets were the ones who gave themselves completely. We never worship a millionaire who had a lot of money and died without being of use to anybody. If you want to live forever, if you want to be immortal, let every minute of your life be useful to the world at large. See that you bring peace and joy to everybody and no harm to anybody. That is the only way; there is no shortcut.

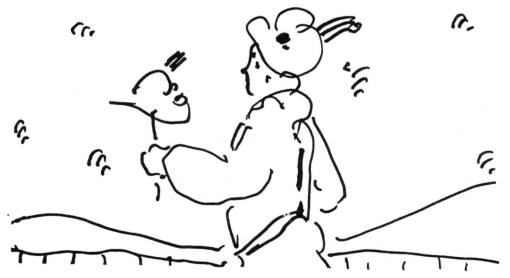

With that outlook on life, the whole world becomes a beautiful Yoga retreat. Then we don't need to retreat from the world, and we don't need to have any treatment because the world will treat us well. Keep these few points in mind and don't worry about theology. "Is there a God here or there? Did I live before? Am I going to live again?" Think of the golden present. The person who thinks of an afterlife wastes this life.

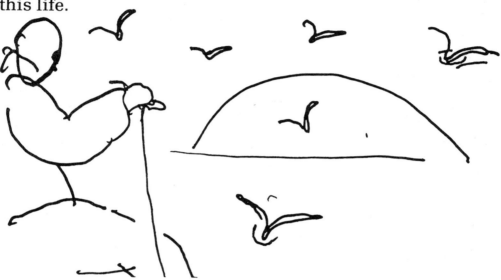

Let the whole world know by your own example that you are something beautiful and divine. Let your actions bring out that cosmic beauty from within. Don't go after cosmetic beauty. Lead a simple life, as natural as possible in dress, food, and behavior. Be like a child.

This will not only take care of you, but your surroundings, your country, and, ultimately, the whole world. Let Yoga reveal to you all of your potential. Go happily, joyfully, peacefully, and share this knowledge, this spirit, and this feeling with the entire world. Share it with all who come close to you—your family, your friends, neighbors, everybody.

Let us all know that there is a vast ocean of consciousness which we call God. Let us not put up barriers or let our ego separate us from it. Open up the heart and say, "Lord I am little. What I know is just a trifle. Please make use of me. Take me as your instrument. Do anything you want. Work through me. It is your business. You created me. You created the world. I don't know why I am here. It's not my business even to ask you. Do anything you want."

Give yourself unto Him. Become humble and selfless and then you will get a glimpse of His joy. If you taste that joy even once in your lifetime, you will know that it is for that joy that we are here.

Integral Yoga means all the Yogas. We approve of all positive approaches. The Integral Yoga Institute doesn't give you one special technique saying, "This is *our* technique." Every positive technique is our technique. This is a way of life. My religion, if you want to call it that, is anything that will make you healthy and happy.

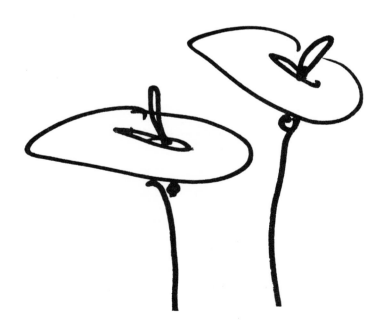

INTEGRAL YOGA INSTITUTES

United States and Canada

Boston, Massachusetts 02115—17 Gloucester Avenue—(617) 536-0444
Dallas, Texas 75205—4012 St. Andrews—(214) 522-4780
Denver, Colorado 80203—857 N. Clarkson Street—(303) 831-8146
Detroit, Michigan 48221—16535 Livernois Avenue—(313) 862-5477
Garfield, New Jersey 07026—5 Clark Street—(201) 546-9666
Los Angeles, California 90046—1427 N. Alta Vista—(213) 876-1272
Montreal, Province of Quebec, H2V 469—5425 Park Avenue—(514) 279-8931
New Britain, Connecticut 06053—198 Gold Street—(203) 224-3220
New Brunswick, New Jersey 08901—103 Church Street—(201) 846-0319
New York, New York 10011—227 West 13th Street—(212) 929-0585
New York, New York 10024—500 West End Avenue—(212) 874-7500
San Antonio, Texas 78212—417 West Craig—(512) 735-1050
San Francisco, California 94110—770 Dolores—(415) 824-9600
Santa Cruz, California 95060—20 Granite Creek Road—(408) 423-8366
Washington, D. C. 20008—2445 Porter Street—(202) 244-5538

India

Coimbatore 18, Tamil Nadu, India—11-D Huzur Road—33220

INTEGRAL YOGA GROUPS

Columbia, Missouri 65201—1503 Wilson Avenue—(314) 449-7066
Iowa City, Iowa 52240—P.O. Box 1244—(319) 326-5702
Kansas City, Missouri 64110—5424 Charlotte—(816) 361-0358

INTEGRAL YOGA TEACHING CENTERS

Tamuning, Guam 96911—P.O. Box 7642
Brookfield, Connecticut 06804—30 Berkshire Drive—(203) 775-4005
Chicago, Illinois 60614—1930 N. Hudson—(312) 327-7877
Dexter, Maine 04930—23 Grove Street—(207) 924-8831
Longwood, Florida 32750—478 East Lake—(305) 831-8149
Paia, Hawaii 96779—P.O. Box 670—(808) 579-9559
Sea Girt, New Jersey 08750—639 Ocean Avenue—(201) 449-5435

ASHRAMS

Satchidananda Ashram-Yogaville East 06259—Box 108 Pomfret Center, Connecticut—(203) 974-1005
Satchidananda Ashram-Yogaville West—1705 San Marcus Pass Road, Santa Barbara, California 93105—(805) 967-3344
Satchidananda Ashram-Arkansas 72632—Box 190 Eureka Springs, Arkansas
Satchidananda Thapovanam—Tekawatte, Tennekumbura, Kandy, Sri Lanka (Ceylon)

Designer's notes

The artwork in this book was generously contributed by Peter Max. These drawings were inspired by Swami Satchidananda and his teachings. Some are reproduced in their original size, while others have been reduced, in entirety or in detail, from larger drawings and limited edition serigraphs. The drawings were created in the period 1966-1977.

The typography for the text is set in Auriga 14 pt. The title and chapter headings are set in Souvenir Light.